# Lecture Notes in Computer Science 2868

Edited by G. Goos, J. Hartmanis, and J. van Leeuwen

# Springer

*Berlin*
*Heidelberg*
*New York*
*Hong Kong*
*London*
*Milan*
*Paris*
*Tokyo*

Petra Perner  Rüdiger Brause
Hermann-Georg Holzhütter (Eds.)

# Medical
# Data Analysis

4th International Symposium, ISMDA 2003
Berlin, Germany, October 9-10, 2003
Proceedings

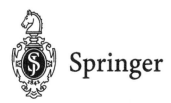

Springer

Series Editors

Gerhard Goos, Karlsruhe University, Germany
Juris Hartmanis, Cornell University, NY, USA
Jan van Leeuwen, Utrecht University, The Netherlands

Volume Editors

Petra Perner
Institute of Computer Vision and Applied Computer Sciences
Körnerstr. 10, 04107 Leipzig, Germany
E-mail: ibaiperner@aol.com

Rüdiger Brause
Johann Wolfgang Goethe-Universität, Institut für Informatik
Robert-Mayer-Str. 11-15, 60054 Frankfurt am Main, Germany
E-mail: brause@informatik.uni-frankfurt.de

Hermann-Georg Holzhütter
Institut für Biochemie, Charité
Campus Mitte, Monbijoustr. 2, 10117 Berlin, Germany
E-mail: hermann-georg.holzhuetter@charite.de

Cataloging-in-Publication Data applied for

A catalog record for this book is available from the Library of Congress.

Bibliographic information published by Die Deutsche Bibliothek
Die Deutsche Bibliothek lists this publication in the Deutsche Nationalbibliografie;
detailed bibliographic data is available in the Internet at <http://dnb.ddb.de>.


CR Subject Classification (1998): H.2.8, I.2, H.3, G.3, I.5.1, I.4, J.3, F.1


ISSN 0302-9743
ISBN 3-540-20282-X Springer-Verlag Berlin Heidelberg New York

Springer-Verlag Berlin Heidelberg New York
a member of BertelsmannSpringer Science+Business Media GmbH

http://www.springer.de

© Springer-Verlag Berlin Heidelberg 2003
Printed in Germany

Typesetting: Camera-ready by author, data conversion by Boller Mediendesign
Printed on acid-free paper      SPIN: 10964101      06/3142      5 4 3 2 1 0

# Preface

The International Symposium on Medical Data Analysis (ISMDA 2003) was the fourth meeting in a series of annual events, organized this year by the Institute of Computer Vision and Applied Computer Sciences (IBaI), Leipzig. The organization of this event was taken over by IBaI on short notice since we wanted to guarantee the smooth continuation of ISMDA. We consider this interdisciplinary research forum as an important platform that helps to drive the development of specific methods of artificial intelligence, signal and image processing, and data mining for medical, health and biological applications. Therefore, the event should continue into the future.

Our special thanks goes to all who contributed to the symposium and made this event successful, in spite of the short time constraints.

The 15 papers in these proceedings cover important topics related to medical models and learning, integration of intelligent analysis methods into medical databases, medical signal and image analysis, and applications of medical diagnostic support systems.

We would like to express our appreciation of the precise and highly professional work of the reviewers. We appreciated the help and understanding of the editorial staff at Springer-Verlag, and in particular Alfred Hofmann, who supported the publication of these proceedings in the LNCS series.

Last, but not least, we wish to thank all the speakers and participants who contributed to the success of the symposium.

October 2003                                                                 Petra Perner

# Organization

## Program Chair

Petra Perner, Leipzig, Germany

## Local Chair

Hermann-Georg Holzhütter, Berlin, Germany

## Program Committee

| | | | |
|---|---|---|---|
| S. Andersen | Denmark | E. Keravnou | Cyprus |
| P. Adlassnig | Austria | J. Kurths | Germany |
| A. Babic | Sweden | M. Kurzynski | Poland |
| R. Brause | Germany | P. Larranaga | Spain |
| R. Bellazzi | Italy | N. Lavrac | Slovenia |
| L. Bobrowski | Poland | R. Lefering | Germany |
| K. Cios | USA | A. Macerata | Italy |
| S. Chillemi | Italy | V. Maojo | Spain |
| L. de Campos | Spain | S. Miksch | Austria |
| G. Dorffner | Austria | A. Neiß | Germany |
| N. Ezquerra | USA | E. Neugebauer | Germany |
| U. Gather | Germany | C. Ohmann | Germany |
| L. Gierl | Germany | L. Pecen | Czech Republic |
| A. Giuliani | Italy | J. Pliskin | Israel |
| O. Hejlesen | Denmark | B. Sierra | Spain |
| H. Holzhütter | Germany | J. Šíma | Czech Republic |
| R. Hovorka | UK | | |

# Table of Contents

## Applications of Medical Diagnostic Support Systems

# Possibility-Probability Relation in Medical Models

A. Bolotin

Department of Epidemiology and Health Sciences Evaluation
Ben-Gurion University of the Negev
P.O. Box 653, Beersheba, 84105, Israel
arkadyv@bgumail.bgu.ac.il

**Abstract.** Medical models based on possibility theory are usually much simpler than those based on probability theory, but they lack foundations. The most foundational question is: How to obtain a possibility distribution for a modeling process? As one of the solutions, a simple framework is proposed built on the conjecture that a probability distribution for an uncertain process can be predicted by the process's possibility distribution. The case of the perfect prediction and the case of possibility and probability distributions related less than perfect (modeling "ideal body weight") are considered in this paper.
*Keywords:* Probability, Possibility theory, Possibility distribution function, Probability density function, Possibilistic modeling in medicine and biology.

## 1 Introduction

The complexity of medical data makes traditional quantitative approaches of analysis inappropriate. There is an unavoidable substantial degree of uncertainty in the description of the behavior of live systems as well as their characteristics. The vagueness in the description of such systems is due to the lack of precise mathematical techniques for dealing with systems comprising a very large number of interacting elements or involving a large number of variables in their decision tree [1].

Usually, the first candidate for the analysis of medical data is the frame-work of probabilities as it is well-known, universally accepted, and built on an axiomatic theory. However, probability cannot easily capture certain situations of interest.

Take, for instance, an example of the bag of color marbles, shown in [2]. Suppose we know 30 marbles are red and we know the remaining 70 are either blue or yellow, although we do not know the exact proportion of blue and yellow. If we are modeling the situation where we pick a ball from the bag at random, we need to assign a probability to three different events: picking up a red ball (red-event), picking up a blue ball (blue-event), and picking up a yellow ball (yellow-event). We can clearly assign a probability of 0.3 to red-event, but there is no clear probability to assign to blue-event or yellow-event.

As one can guess, the situation like this (in which we just cannot clearly assign probabilities to certain events) is quite often in modeling uncertain medical knowledge. To offer an alternative to probability theory, other uncertainty frameworks have been proposed. Among them, possibility theory (as one of the major non-probabilistic the-

P. Perner et al. (Eds.): ISMDA 2003, LNCS 2868, pp. 1-8, 2003.

ory of uncertainty) has gained much attention [3-9]. Such attention can be explained mostly by the fact that operations between possibilistic elements are usually much simpler than those between probabilistic elements. As a result, models based on possibility distributions usually prove to be simpler than those built on probability distributions [10-11].

On the other hand, in modeling uncertainty with possibility theory the foundational question is: *How to obtain a possibility distribution for a given process/system* [12]? In principle, we have two choices: We can draw off a possibility distribution from a theory, or we can simply extract possibilities from an experiment by measurements.

The first choice is realized in physical science applications. Take, for example, quantum mechanics. Here, the central mathematical element is the wave function $\Psi(x)$, which represents all the possibilities $\mu(x)$ that can happen to an observed process $x$ when it interacts with an observing device (a measuring device):

$$\mu(x) = \frac{|\Psi(x)|}{\sup|\Psi(x)|} \quad .$$
(1)

The wave function is calculated theoretically via the Schrödinger wave equation for any moment between the time the observed process $x$ leaves the region of preparation and the time that it interacts with the measuring device.

Such theoretical way (to obtain a possibility distribution for an observed process $x$) is unacceptable in medical modeling just because a precise model may not exist for biological processes/systems (or it may be too difficult to model).

At the same time, to obtain possibilities empirically (i.e. through measurements) one needs to know the exact form of relation between possibility and probability distributions. This knowledge is essential because *possibility distributions cannot be measured directly* [13].

Consider, for example, $\mu(x')$ - the possibility to classify the income $\$ x'$ as "fair". Before we ask an individual from the study group the question "Can you classify the income $\$ x'$ as "fair"?", we have two possibilities:

$$\begin{cases} \text{Pos}_{\text{Yes}} = \mu(x') \\ \text{Pos}_{\text{No}} = 1 - \mu(x') \end{cases} ;$$
(2)

where $\text{Pos}_{\text{Yes}}$ is the possibility that the individual will answer yes, and $\text{Pos}_{\text{No}}$ is the possibility that the individual will answer no. Once, however, the individual answers this question, the possibilities $\text{Pos}_{\text{Yes}}$ and $\text{Pos}_{\text{No}}$ abruptly discontinuously change: one of the possibilities ceases to exist (i.e. becomes 0), while the other possibility actualizes (i.e. turns to 1). Thus, what we really get measuring $\mu(x')$ is the proportion of people $p(x')\Delta x$ who classify $x'$ as "fair income" (where $p(x)$ is the corresponding probability distribution).

In our paper we will concentrate on the study of the relation between possibility and probability distributions in medical models. We will present this relation in the form of a simple framework basing generally on intuitive argumentation.

## 2  Conjecture of the Prediction

We will begin with a summary of notations from possibility and probability theories.

**1.** To describe values of an uncertain process $x$ we can define a probability distribution $p(x)$: $p(x')dx$ gives the probability to find $x'$ in the interval $(x', x' + dx)$. The function $p(x)$ meets the following key condition called *the probabilistic normalization*:

$$\int_X p(x)\, dx = 1 \quad , \tag{3}$$

where $X$ is the universe of $x$.

**2.** To describe the same uncertain process we can also define a possibility distribution $\mu(x)$: $\mu(x')$ gives the degree of possibility that $x = x'$ with the following conventions:

(1) $\mu(x') = 0$ means that the event $x = x'$ is impossible,

(2) $\mu(x') = 1$ means that the event $x = x'$ is possible without any restriction.

Considering the assumption that $X$ contains all possible values of $x$, there must at least one $x' \in X$ such that $\mu(x') = 1$. We can formulate this as *the possibilistic normalization*:

$$\sup_{x \in X} \mu(x) = 1 \quad . \tag{4}$$

**3.** It is obvious that if the event is not possible, it cannot be probable. Hence, the first thing we can say about the relation between possibility and probability distributions is that

$$p(x_o) = 0 \quad \text{if } \mu(x_o) = 0 \quad . \tag{5}$$

**4.** Besides, we can assert that out of two events that one is less probable which is less possible:

$$p(x_1) < p(x_2) \quad \text{if } \mu(x_1) < \mu(x_2) \quad . \tag{6}$$

That is, the value of the function $p(x)$ is decreasing if the function $\mu(x)$ is going down, and the function $p(x)$ is going up if the $\mu(x)$ is rising.

**5.** Considering (5) and (6) together, we can say that a probability distribution $p(x)$ for a process $x$ can be predicted by the process's possibility distribution $\mu(x)$. We will call the last assertion *the conjecture of the prediction* and put it as a base for our framework.

## 3  Case of the Perfect Prediction

In the extreme case of the perfect prediction we have:

$$p(x) = F[\mu(x)] \quad , \tag{7}$$

where $F$ is a function connecting $\mu$ values with $p$ values. The function $F$ meets all the following conditions:

(1) when $x = x_o$ represents an impossible event, the $F$ must equal zero

$$F[0] = 0 \quad ; \tag{8}$$

(2) the $F$ is a non-negative function

$$F[\mu(x)] \geq 0 \quad ; \tag{9}$$

(3) the integral of $F$ over $X$ has to be equal to 1

$$\int_X F[\mu(x)]dx = 1 \quad . \tag{10}$$

The perfect prediction takes place in quantum mechanics. Indeed, according to the main postulate of quantum mechanics [14-19], the probabilities at a given time(s) of each of the possibilities represented by wave function $\Psi(x)$ are:

$$p(x) = |\Psi(x)|^2 \quad . \tag{11}$$

Combining (11) with the definition (1) we find

$$p(x) = \text{const} \cdot \mu^2(x) \quad . \tag{12}$$

## 4  Case of the Less-than-Perfect Prediction

If a possibility distribution $\mu(x)$ cannot be derived from a theory, or may be determined only subjectively, or from empirical evidence, this function $\mu(x)$ cannot perfectly predict a probability distribution $p(x)$. The prediction will be with errors included in the predicted values for $p(x)$. When these errors are, in some sense small, we have a *case of the less-than perfect prediction.*

**1.** Assume we study the self-perception of the body weight in some particular population. Let $x$ represent the weight. We want to know the $\mu(x)$ - the degree of possibility that people of that population will consider $x$ as "ideal weight". Since we have no theory, any reasonable function $\mu(x)$ can be used as a model for "ideal weight".

**2.** Let $M$ be a set of the $\mu(x)$ functions such that each $\mu(x)$ of $M$ can be used as a model for "ideal weight", and let $\rho$ be a probability of a function $\mu(x)$ being randomly selected from the set $M$. By analogy with the case of perfect prediction, we will assert that

$$p(x) = F[\overline{\mu}(x)] \quad , \tag{13}$$

$\overline{\mu}(x)$ is the mean possibility distribution for "ideal weight"; $p(x)$ gives the proportion of people who will classify the weight $x$ as "ideal"; $F$ is the function connecting $\overline{\mu}$ values with $p$ values, the $F$ meets all the conditions (8)-(10).

**3.** Let $\Delta\mu(x)$ denote a random variable such that

$$\mu(x) = \overline{\mu}(x) - \Delta\mu(x) \quad . \tag{14}$$

Assume that values of the $\Delta\mu(x)$ are very small, that is, $\overline{\mu}(x) \gg \Delta\mu(x)$. Then we can expand the function $F[\overline{\mu}(x)]$ in a power series of the variable $\Delta\mu(x)$ :

$$F[\overline{\mu}(x)] = F[\mu(x)] + \sum_{j=1} \frac{1}{j!} \frac{\partial^j F}{\partial\mu^j} [\Delta\mu(x)]^j \quad . \tag{15}$$

On substituting this expansion in (13), and neglecting terms above the second order of $\Delta\mu(x)$, we have

$$p(x) \cong F[\mu(x)] + \frac{\partial F}{\partial\mu} \Delta\mu(x) \quad . \tag{16}$$

**4.** Suppose, conducting our statistical survey we ask people of the study population to answer only by yes or no to the series of questions "Can you classify the weight $x_i$ as "ideal"?" (where $x_i$ denotes one of the $N$ preselected $x$ values), and come up with the frequencies of positive answers ( $p_1, \ldots p_i, \ldots p_N$ ). Let the particular function $\mu(x)$ be selected, and $N$ calculations of the $\mu(x)$ be made, corresponding to the preselected $x$ values. Then we get the results ( $x_1, \mu_1, p_1$ ), ..., ( $x_N, \mu_N, p_N$ ), where

$$p_i = F[\mu_i] + \varepsilon_i \quad ; \tag{17}$$

$\varepsilon_i$ denotes the value $(\partial F/\partial \mu) \cdot \Delta\mu(x)$ at $x_i$; ( $\varepsilon_1, \ldots, \varepsilon_N$ ) has a multivariate normal distribution with mean vector $(0,0,\ldots,0)$.

**5.** Consider the case when we can simplify the equation (17) by expanding the $F[\mu_i]$ into a power series of the $\mu_i$ :

$$p_i = \sum_{k=1} b_k \mu_i^k + \varepsilon_i \quad . \tag{18}$$

**6.** As a set $M$ (set of the $\mu$ functions for "ideal weight" modeling) we can use, for example, the following class of symmetrical membership functions [20]:

$$\mu(x) = \begin{cases} 0 & \text{for } x \leq \alpha + \Delta\alpha \\ c \cdot \exp\left[-\dfrac{(1+\Delta\gamma)^{-1}}{(x-\alpha-\Delta\alpha)(\beta+\Delta\beta-x)}\right] & \text{for } \alpha+\Delta\alpha < x < \beta+\Delta\beta \quad ; \\ 0 & \text{for } x \geq \beta+\Delta\beta \end{cases} \tag{19}$$

$\alpha$ and $\beta$ represent the lower and upper bounds for the "ideal weight" interval respectively; $\Delta\alpha$, $\Delta\beta$ and $\Delta\gamma$ denote small random variables (small "uncertainties") such that $\alpha \gg \Delta\alpha$, $\beta \gg \Delta\beta$ and $1 \gg \Delta\gamma$; $c$ is the possibilistic normalization coefficient. Changing the $\Delta\alpha$ and $\Delta\beta$ changes the interval ( $\alpha, \beta$ ) in which the function $\mu(x)$ differs from zero. Changing the $\Delta\gamma$ makes the shape of the $\mu(x)$ wider (if $\Delta\gamma > 0$) or smaller (if $\Delta\gamma < 0$). The class of the normalized functions (19) is plotted in Fig. 1.

On substituting (19) in (18), we receive for the interval $\alpha < x < \beta$ :

$$p_i = cb_1 \exp\left[-\frac{1}{(x_i-\alpha)(\beta-x_i)}\right] + c^2 b_2 \exp\left[-\frac{2}{(x_i-\alpha)(\beta-x_i)}\right] + \\ + c^3 b_3 \exp\left[-\frac{3}{(x_i-\alpha)(\beta-x_i)}\right] + \ldots + \varepsilon_i \tag{20}$$

where $c = \exp[4/(\beta-\alpha)^2]$.

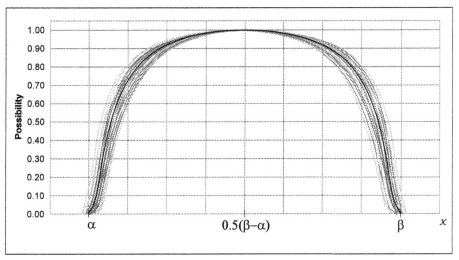

**Fig. 1.** The class of the $\mu$ functions for "ideal weight" modeling.

(In the graph each line was generated using a different set of the uncertainties $\Delta\alpha$, $\Delta\beta$, $\Delta\gamma$ ; the line's color approximately correlates with the value of the uncertainties: the greater the uncertainties, the smaller percent of black was used drawing the line.)

It is seen, that (20) is the exponential regression equation for estimating the combination of the $b$ coefficients and the parameters $\alpha$ and $\beta$. Thus, as one can conclude, the problem of determination of the possibility distribution from empirical frequencies may be reduced to the regression problem.

# References

[1] M. Abbod, D. von Keyserlingk, D. Linkens, M. Mahfouf (2001). Survey of utilization of fuzzy technology in Medicine and Healthcare. *Fuzzy Sets and Systems* **120** 331–349, 2001

[2] J. Halpern and R. Pucella (2002). Logic for Reasoning about Upper Probabilities. *Articial Intelligence Research* **17** 57-81, 2002.

[3] D. Dubois and H. Prade (1988). An introduction to possibilistic and fuzzy logics. In *Non-Standard Logics for Automated Reasoning*, (Edited by P. Smets, A. Mamdani, D. Dubois, H. Prade), Academic Press, London, pp. 287-315, 1988.

[4] S. Lapointe and B. Bobée (2000). Revision of possibility distributions: A Bayesian inference patern. *Fuzzy sets and systems* **116** 119-140, 2000.

[5] L. Zadeh (1978). Fuzzy sets as a basis for theory of possibility. *Fuzzy sets and systems* **1** 3-28, 1978.

[6] L. Zadeh (1978). PRUF – a measuring representation language for natural languages. *Internat. J. Man-Machine Studies* **10** 395-460, 1978.

[7]  L. Zadeh (1981). Possibility theory and soft data analysis, In *Mathematical Frontiers of the Social and Policy Sciences*, (Edited by L. Cobb, R. Thrall), pp. 69-129. Westview Press. Boulder CO, 1981.

[8]  G. Klir (2000). On fuzzy-set interpretation of possibility theory. *Fuzzy sets and systems* **108** 263-273, 2000.

[9]  P. Walley (1996). Measures of uncertainty in expert systems. *Artificial Intelligence* **83** 1-58, 1996.

[10]  G. de Cooman (1997). Possibility Theory I: The measure- and integral-theoretic groundwork. *Internat. J. General Systems* **25** 291-323, 1997.

[11]  H. Janssen, G. de Cooman, E. Kerre (1999). A Daniel-Kolmogorov theorem for supremum preserving upper probabilities. *Fuzzy sets and systems* **102** 429-444, 1999.

[12]  H. Nguyen (1997). Fuzzy sets and probability. *Fuzzy sets and systems* **90** 129-132, 1997.

[13]  A. Bolotin (2001). A Generalized Uncertainty Function and Fuzzy Modeling, In *J. Crespo, V. Maojo, and F. Martin (Eds.): ISMDA 2001, LNCS 2199*, pp. 75-80. Springer-Verlag Berlin Heidelberg, 2001.

[14]  J. Mehra and H. Rechenberg (2001). *The Historical Development of Quantum Theory*, Springer Verlag, 2001.

[15]  H. Strap (1972). The Copenhagen Interpretation and the Nature of Space-Time. *American Journal of Physics*, **40** 1098, 1972.

[16]  W. Heisenberg (1958). *Physics and Philosophy*, Harper Torch Books, New York, 1958.

[17]  J. von Neumann (1955). *The Mathematical Foundations of Quantum Mechanics*, Princeton University Press, Princeton, 1955.

[18]  J. Bell (1981). Bertlmann's socks and the nature of reality. *J. Phys. C* **2** 41–62, 1981.

[19]  J. Dalibard and J.-L. Basdevant (2000). *The Quantum Mechanics Solver: How to Apply Quantum Theory to Modern Physics (Advanced Texts in Physics)*, Springer Verlag, 2000.

[20]  A. Grauel and L. Ludwig (1999). Construction of differentiable membership functions. *Fuzzy sets and systems* **101** 219-225, 1999.

# How Exactly Do We Know Inheritance Parameters?

Karl-Ernst Biebler, Bernd Jäger, Michael Wodny

Institute of Biometry and Medical Informatics
Ernst-Moritz-Arndt-University
Rathenaustraße 48
D-19487 Greifswald, Germany
biebler@biometrie.uni-greifswald.de

**Abstract.** There are different concepts to quantify the information contained in a data set. The classic result is from R.A.Fisher: Regarding a sample over a random variable. The Fisher-Information is defined under certain assumptions as the inverse of the Rao-Cramer barrier in the well known inequality of the same name. The Fisher-Informations are considered for the simplest genetic models of intheritance. This applies to medically relevant ranges of the inheritance model parameter and large data sets. The results are compared with exact calculations.

## 1 Introduction

The estimation of allele probabilities is essential for the closer quantitative identification of inheritance. It requires the probabilistic formulation of the applied model of inheritance. Allele probabilities become the parameters in the probabilistic model and will be estimated by maximum-likelihood methods ([1], [2]).

Properties of these estimators are of asymptotic character mostly. Unbiasedness and efficiency can be proven in special cases. This is the background for approximate sample size and confidence interval calculations in the context of population based genetic investigations. Approximate calculations are too inaccurate for the simplest model of inheritance, large data sets and genetically relevant order of magnitude of the parameters. An exact method of sample size calculation is recommended.

As a conclusion, geneticists have to quantify the methodological bias of their investigations carefully.

The computations were carried out in both MATHEMATICA and SAS with numerically identical results.

## 2 The One-Locus-Two-Allele Model

A two-allele model without any dominance relations is described by the probabilistic model

P. Perner et al. (Eds.): ISMDA 2003, LNCS 2868, pp. 9-14, 2003.
© Springer-Verlag Berlin Heidelberg 2003

$$M_1 = \begin{bmatrix} \{(A_1 A_1),(A_1 A_2),(A_2 A_2)\}\,; \\ P(A_1 A_1) = p^2,\, P(A_1 A_2) = 2p(1-p),\, P(A_2 A_2) = (1-p)^2 \end{bmatrix}.$$

The phenotypes observed are exactly the genotypes $A_i A_j$. The maximum-likelihood estimator related to $M_1$ is the so called gene counting method,

$$\hat{p}_1 = (2N(A_1 A_1) + N(A_1 A_2))/(2N).$$

The random variable $2N\,\hat{p}_1$ describes the number of alleles of type $A_1$ in a sample of size $2N$. It is binomially distributed with parameters $2N$ and $p$. The estimator $\hat{p}_1$ is unbiased,

$$E(\hat{p}_1) = \frac{1}{2N} E(2N\hat{p}_1) = \frac{1}{2N} 2Np = p.$$

Its variance

$$V(\hat{p}_1) = \frac{1}{(2N)^2} V(2N\hat{p}_1) = \frac{1}{(2N)^2} 2Np(1-p) = \frac{p(1-p)}{2N}$$

coincides with the inverse of the Fisher-Information. Due to the Rao-Cramer ine-quali-ty, the maximum-likelihood estimator (MLE ) $\hat{p}_1$ is efficient [1].
If $A_1$ is the dominating allele, we obtain

$$M_2 = \begin{bmatrix} \{(A_1 A_1, A_1 A_2),(A_2 A_2)\}\,; \\ P(A_1 A_1, A_1 A_2) = 1-(1-p)^2,\, P(A_2 A_2) = (1-p)^2 \end{bmatrix}$$

and the MLE

$$\hat{p}_2 = 1 - \sqrt{\frac{N(A_2 A_2)}{N}}.$$

If $A_2$ is the dominating allele, the probabilistic model

$$M_3 = \begin{bmatrix} \{(A_1 A_1),(A_1 A_2, A_2 A_2)\}\,; \\ P(A_1 A_1) = p^2,\, P(A_1 A_2, A_2 A_2) = 1-p^2 \end{bmatrix}$$

gives the MLE

$$\hat{p}_3 = \sqrt{\frac{N(A_1 A_1)}{N}}.$$

Both $\hat{p}_2$ and $\hat{p}_3$ are neither unbiased nor effective estimators of $p$.

The random variables $N(1-\hat{p}_2)^2$ and $N(\hat{p}_3)^2$ are binomially distributed with pa-rameters $N$, $(1-p)^2$ and $N$, $p^2$, respectively. Due to the statistical estimation theory, the estimators $\hat{p}_2$ and $\hat{p}_3$ are both asymptotically efficient and asymptotically unbiased. Their asymptotic variances (Rao-Cramer inequality) are calculated from the related Fisher-Informations as

$$V_{asymp}(\hat{p}_2) = \frac{2p - p^2}{4N} \qquad \text{and} \qquad V_{asymp}(\hat{p}_3) = \frac{1 - p^2}{4N}.$$

## 3 Allele Probability Estimation and Related Sample Sizes

At the simple example of the calculation of phenotype probabilities for phenylketonuria (PKU) from population data it will demonstrated that approximate methods to noteworthy faults can lead. The model of inheritance of the PKU is $M_3$. The data mining operation $\hat{p} = \hat{p}_3$ is a random variable. It shall be characterized by the analysis of confidence intervals statistically.

There are three possibilities for the calculation of these confidence intervals:

**Method 1.** One calculates they exactly with respect to the binomial distribution with the parameters $N$ and $p^2$.

**Method 2.** One calculates they asymptotically according to the limit theorem of Laplace under reference to the normal distribution with the expectation $Np^2$ and the variance $Np^2(1-p^2)$.

**Method 3.** One calculates they asymptotically according to the limit theorem from the theory of maximum-likelihood estimations under reference to the normal distribution with the expectation value $p$ and the variance $V_{asymp}$.

The exact calculation of confidence intervals for the parameter $p$ of a Binomial distribution is possible with the help of incomplete Beta functions $I_p$, ([3]),

$$P(X \geq k) = \sum_{j=k}^{n} \binom{n}{k} p^k (1-p)^{n-k}$$

$$= I_p(k, n-k+1)$$

$$= \frac{\int_0^p t^k (1-t)^{n-k} \, dt}{\int_0^1 t^k (1-t)^{n-k} \, dt} = \frac{B_p(k, n-k+1)}{B(k, n-k+1)}.$$

The calculation methods yield different confidence intervals for $p$. For an example the Figures 1, 2 and 3 illustrate these differences.

## 4 Sample Size Calculation for PKU

We discuss now the sample size calculations for predefined length of confidence intervals for the incidence $p^2$ of the PKU. They have practical interest for the planning of clinical or epidemiological studies and for the evaluation of population genetic data and are based on the Methods 1 and 2 mentioned above. The calculations were carried out in SAS [4] and in MATHEMATICA. The programs are sent upon request.

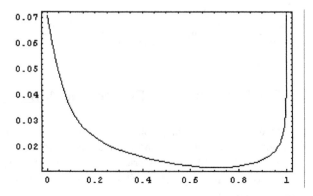

**Fig. 1.** Difference of the exact length and the asymptotic Laplace-calculated length of the 0.95-confidence interval as a function of $p$, $N = 50$.

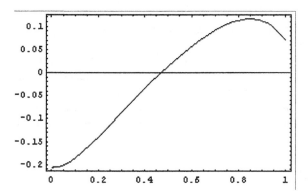

**Fig. 2.** Difference of the exact length and the asymptotic due to maximum-likelihood calculated length of the 0.95-confidence interval as a function of $p$, $N = 50$.

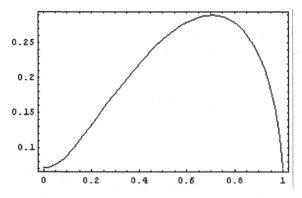

**Fig. 3.** Exact length of the 0.95-confidence interval as a function of $p$, $N = 50$.

The confidence level is 0.95 in the following, the length $B$ of the confidence interval has to be fixed. For given values of $p$, necessary sample sizes are calculable from
the probability distributions of $\hat{p}$.

PKU is one of the most frequent hereditary diseases. For a certain population the
allele probability of PKU is supposed as $p = 0.01$. This is a realistic order of magnitude. The incidence (phenotype probability) for "ill" then is $p^2 = 0.0001$.
Figure 4 shows the length of the 0.95-confidence interval of the phenotype probabilities as a function of the sample size $N$.
For $B = p^2 = 0.0001$ arises a necessary sample size as $N = 173\ 146$ (Method 1). The
approximate Method 2 yields $N = 153\ 649$.

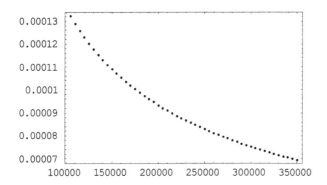

**Fig. 4.** Exact length of the 0.95-confidence interval of p, as a function of sample size
N, calculated in the neighbourhood of p= 0.0001

For $B$ equals 10% of the incidence $p^2 = 0.0001$ is the result (Method 1) approximately
$N = 15\ 570\ 000$.
   The calculation of incidences for hereditary diseases from population samples requires exceptionally big sample sizes. Are such examinations possible?
It has to be taken from the table 6.3 into [5] that all 886287 newborn children of East-
ern Germany (former DDR, about 17 million inhabitants) then were tested on PKU in
the time period 1969 to 1974. One found 95 cases at it. This yields an incidence of
0.000 107 and an exact calculated 0.95-confidence interval [0,000 087 ; 0.000131]
for this five years time period. The length of this confidence interval is 41% of the
stated incidence.
It is not possible to improve the precision of the incidence for the examined population !
Consider now the estimation of the allele probability $p$. For $p = 0.01$ and the same
length $B$ of the 0.95-onfidence interval one gets with Method 3 a necessary sample
size $N = 38413$. The exact Method 1 yields $N = 45\ 865$ here.

## 5  Conclusions

If for a model of inheritance all genotypes are completely observable, the calculation of the allele probabilities can be carried out according to the gene counting method. It is an unbiased and effective estimator. Approximate (regarding the Fisher-Information) and exactly calculated sample sizes concerning confidence estimations of allele probabilities agree well.

These statements are no longer correct if you evaluate phenotype data. Already for the very simple model of inheritance $M_3$ for the PKU there are considerable differences between the approximate and the exact calculated sample sizes. Consequently, the approximate calculation methods should not be used longer.

The information content has to be carefully judged also for large population genetic data sets. As seen from the PKU population data, exactly calculated confidence intervals may serve for that. The precision of incidence estimates is not high also for frequent hereditary diseases (e.g. PKU). Geneticists must accept an inaccuracy of their findings.

## References

1. Biebler, K.E., Jäger, B.: Punkt- und Konfidenzschätzungen von Allelwahrscheinlichkeiten.. In: Simianer, H.:Biometrische Aspekte der Genomanalyse. GinkgoPark Mediengesellschaft,. Berlin.(1996) 19 - 42
2. Encyclopedia of Biostatistics. Wiley, Chichester (1998) 1609 - 1613
3. Johnson, N.L., Kotz, S., Kemp, A.W.: Univariate discrete distributions. 2 nd edn.. John Wiley & Sons Inc. (1992)
4. Daly, L.: Simple SAS macros for the calculation of exact binomial and Poisson confidence limits. Comput. Biol. Med.Vol.22. No 5. (1992) 351-361
5. Vogel, F., Motulsky, A.G.: Human Genetics. Springer-Verlag, Berlin Heidelberg New York.. (1979)

# Tuning of Diagnosis Support Rules through Visualizing Data Transformations[1]

Leon Bobrowski[a,b], Magda Topczewska[a]

[a]Faculty of Computer Science, Technical University of Białystok

[b]Institute of Biocybernetics and Biomedical Engineering, PAS, Warsaw

**Abstract.** Medical diagnosis support is often based on the case based reasoning (CBR) scheme. In accordance with this scheme, the record of a new patient is compared with similar records of previous patients with confirmed diagnosis. Such scheme has been implemented among others in the Hepar system, which comprises a hepathological database and a variety of procedures that aim at data analysis and the support of diagnosis. The diagnosis support rules of this system are based on the visualizing data transformations combined with the nearest neighbors technique. The applied transformations of data sets allow not only for data visualization but also for modifications of the distance or similarity measures used in the nearest neighbors technique. In this way, similarity measures can be induced from data sets.

*Keywords: diagnosis support rules, data visualization, case based reasoning*


## 1. Introduction

Computer-based systems supporting a medical diagnosis can be based on a variety of principles. One of the most fundamental scheme is the case based reasoning (CBR). The CBR scheme is a problem-solving paradigm which utilizes specific knowledge of previously experienced situations (cases) stored in a "Case Base" [1]. A new diagnostic problem is solved by finding and reusing similar past cases.

A basic question in applying the case based reasoning scheme is how to choose the similarity measure between the patients or, more generally, between the cases stored in the database. The nearest neighbors (K-NN) method of classification is being used as the CBR scheme in the diagnosis support systems [2]. Generally, the nearest neighbors classification or diagnostic rules are based on the comparisons of a newly

---

[1] This work was partially supported by the grant W/II/1/2003 from the Białystok University of Technology and by the grant 16/St/2003 from the Institute of Biocybernetics and Biomedical Engineering PAS.

P. Perner et al. (Eds.): ISMDA 2003, LNCS 2868, pp. 15-22, 2003.

object with the most close or similar objects that have been previously classified. A common practice is to use the Euclidean distance between numerical representations of the patients records in the database, as the measure of similarity between the patients. It is known, that in many situations the Euclidean distance is not an adequate measure of similarity. In some situations, the Euclidean distance could be even difficult to determine.

We are exploring here the possibility of improving the similarity measure between the patients based on the Euclidean distance. For this purpose, we are combining the nearest neighbors technique with the visualizing data transformations. In other words, we propose to use the Euclidean distance or other measures of similarity to the objects represented on the visualizing plane. Such scheme has been implemented in the computer system Hepar [3]. The system comprises Hepar of a hepathological database and a variety of procedures that aim at data analysis and the support of diagnosis. The database of the system contains the results of medical findings for more than 800 patients from the Gastroenterological Clinic of the Institute of Food and Feeding in Warsaw. Each case is described by about 200 medical findings and histopathologically verified diagnosis. The patients from this database have been classified by clinicians into about 20 liver diseases.

The visualizing plane could result from the linear or nonlinear transformations of data sets. We design the visualizing transformations through minimization of the convex and piecewise linear (CPL) criterion function. The perceptron criterion function which is linked to the beginning of the theory of neural network belongs to the CPL family. We have been developing recently the dipolar and the differential criterion functions which also belongs to the CPL family [4], [5]. The dipolar approach allows to design the visualizing planes with a good separability between diseases.

## 2. Linear Transformations of the Learning Sets

Let us assume, that the records of a clinical database are represented as the n-dimensional feature vectors $x = [x1,......,xn]T$. The component (feature) $xji$ of the vector $xj$ is a numerical result of the i-th diagnostic examination ($i =1,...,n$) of a given patient $Oj$ ($j = 1,......, m$). The medical feature vectors $xj$ are often of a mixed type, because they contain both symptoms and signs ($xi \in \{0,1\}$) as well as results of laboratory tests ($xi \in R$) performed on a given patient.

The feature vectors $xj(k)$ representing records of a clinical database are usually labelled in accordance with the clinical diagnosis $\omega k$ ($k =1,.....,K$). The symbol $xj(k)$ means, that the j-th patient $Oj$ has been linked by clinicians to the k-th disease $\omega k$. For example, in the case of the Hepar system, the symbol $\omega k$ indicates one of the possible liver disorders [3]. Each diagnosis in Hepar has been histopatologically verified by clinicians. Based on the diagnosis $\omega k$, the labelled feature vectors $xj(k)$ have been divided into the learning sets $Ck$:

$$Ck = \{xj(k)\} \quad (j \in Ik) \tag{1}$$

where $Ik$ is the set of the indices j of the vectors $xj(k)$ related to the class $\omega k$.

Let us consider the linear transformations of the vectors xj(k) on the plane. The vectors xj(k) are transformed into the points yj(k) on the visualizing plane in the following manner:

$$yj(k) = [yj1(k), yj2(k)]T = [<w1,xj(k)>,<w2,xj(k)>]T \qquad (2)$$

where wi= [wi1,.....,win]T∈ Rn (i =1,2) are the weight vectors, and <wi,x> are the inner products. The scatterplots or, in other words, the maps of data sets are generated as the result of the visualisation of the transformed points yj(k). If the vectors wi are orthogonal (<w1,w2> = 0) and have the unit length (<w1,w1> = (<w2,w2> = 0) then the transformations (2) describes the projection of the feature vectors xj(k) on the visualizing plane  P(w1,w2) = {x: x = α1 w1+ α2 w2, gdzie αi ∈R1}.

The parameter vectors wi of the transformation (2) can be estimated from the learning sets Ck (1) in a variety of ways. The most popular estimation methods  are based on solving of the eigenvalue problem with a symmetric, covariance-like matrix Σ [6]. In our approach, the optimal value of the parameter vectors w1 and w2 (2) is found through minimisation of the convex and piecewise-linear criterion functions defined on the so called dipoles [4].

Definition 1: The pair {xj(k), xj'(k)} (j<j') of the feature vectors xj(k) and xj(k) constitutes the clear dipole, if these vectors belong to the same category ωk. Two feature vectors xjk) and xj'(k') from different categories ωk and ωk' constitute a mixed dipole{xj(k), xj'(k')}

Definition 2: The dipole {xj(k), x j'(k')} (j<j') is positively oriented if and only if for the given weight vector w* the product <w*, xj(k)- xj'(k')> is positive. The dipole {xj(k), x j'(k')} (j<j') is negatively oriented if and only if <w*, xj(k)- xj'(k')> < 0.

The dipoles {xj(k), xj'(k')}of the length δx(j,j') are transformed by (2) into the dipoles {yj(k), yj'(k')}- the pairs of the points yj(k) and  yj'(k) situated on the plane in the Euclidean distance δy(j,j'), where

$$δx2(j,j') = < xj(k)- xj'(k'), xj(k)- xj'(k')> \qquad (3)$$
and
$$δy2(j,j') = < yj(k)- yj'(k'), yj(k)- yj'(k')> \qquad (4)$$

We are interested in designing of such visualizing transformations (2) which result in short clear dipoles {yj(k), yj'(k)} and long mixed dipoles{yj(k), yj'(k')}. Let us remark, that the transformation (2) which fulfils the above postulate can give a good separability of the classes ωk on the visualizing plane. Such separability postulate can be implemented by using of adequately tailored differential CPL criterion function, which is defined below [4], [5].

## 3. Differential Criterion Function

Let us define the CPL penalty functions φjj'+(w) and φjj'-(w) based on the differences xj(k) - xj'(k') of the feature vectors xj(k) and xj'(k'):

$$\phi jj'+(w) = \begin{cases} 0 & \text{if } <w, xj(k)- xj'(k')> < ajj' \\ -aij' + <w, xj(k)- xj'(k') > & \text{if } <w, xj(k)- xj'(k')> > ajj' \end{cases} \quad (5)$$

$$\phi jj'-(w) = \begin{cases} 0 & \text{if } <w, xj(k)- xj'(k')> > bjj' \\ bij' - <w, xj(k)- xj'(k') > & \text{if } <w, xj(k)- xj'(k') > < bjj' \end{cases} \quad (6)$$

where $aij'$ and $bij'$ are the margins related to the dipole $\{xj(k), xj'(k')\}$.

The differential criterion function $\Phi(w)$ is defined as the sum of the piecewise linear and convex penalty functions $\phi jj'+(w)$ and $\phi jj'-(w)$ multiplied by the nonnegative coefficients $\gamma jj'$:

$$\Phi(w) = \Sigma \; \gamma jj' \; \phi jj'+(w) + \Sigma \; \gamma jj' \; \phi jj'-(w) + \Sigma \; \gamma jj' \; (\phi jj'+(w) + \phi jj'-(w)) \quad (7)$$
$$(j,j') \in \text{Im} + (j,j') \in \text{Im-} (j,j') \in \text{Ic}$$

where the coefficient $\gamma jj' \geq 0$ determines a price of the dipole $\{xj(k),xj'(k')\}$. The symbol Im+ stands for the set of the indices $(j, j')$ of the mixed and positively oriented dipoles (Def. 2).. The symbol Im- means the set of the indices $(j, j')$ of the mixed and negatively oriented dipoles (Im+∩ Im- = $\varnothing$). Ic is the subset of indices $(j,j')$ of the clear dipoles $\{xj(k),xj'(k)\}$.

It has been proved, that $\Phi(v)$ (6) is the convex and piecewise linear (CPL) function. The basis exchange algorithms, similar to linear programming allow to find a minimum of such type of functions efficiently, even in the case of large, multidimensional learning sets Ck [7]:

$$\Phi^* = \Phi(w^*) = \min \Phi(w) \quad (8)$$

The optimal parameter vectors $w^*$ and the minimal values $\Phi^*$ of the criterion function $\Phi(w)$ (7) can be applied to a variety of problems. In particular, the vectors wi defining the transformations (2) can be found by the minimisation of the function $\Phi i(w)$. The minimization of the differential criterion function $\Phi(w)$ (7) gives possibility for shortening the clear dipoles $\{yj(k), yj'(k)\}$ and for lengthening the mixed dipoles.

## 4. The Nearest Neighbors Rules

The nearest neighbours diagnosis support rules are based on the distances $\delta(x0,xj(k))$ between the feature vector x0 of a newly diagnosed patient and the labelled vectors xj(k) from the clinical database. Let us assume for a moment, that the labelled feature vectors xj(k) could be ranked in respect to the distances $\delta(x0,xj(k))$ between the vectors x0 and xj(k):

$$(\forall i \in \{1,....,m-1\}) \; \delta(x0,xj(i)) \leq \delta(x0,xj(i+1)) \quad (9)$$

The ball Bx(x0,K) centred in x0 and containing exactly K ranked vectors xj(k) can be defined:

$$Bx(x0,K) = \{xj(k): \delta(x0,xj(i)) \leq \delta(x0,xj(K)) \tag{10}$$

In accordance with the K-nearest neighbours (K-NN) rule, the object x0 is allocated into this class ωk where most of the labelled feature vectors xj(k) from the ball Bx(x0,K) belong [2]:

$$if \ (\forall l \in \{1,...,K\}) \ nk \geq nl \ \ then \ \ x0 \in \omega k \tag{11}$$

where nk is the number of the vectors xj(k) from the set Ck (1) contained in the ball Bx(x0,K).

The Euclidean distance $\delta E(x0,xj(k)) = <x0 - xj(k), x0- xj(k)>$ (3) is commonly used in the nearest neighbours classification or in diagnosis support rules. The quality of such rules can be often improved by optimisation of the neighbours number K and the distance function $\delta(x0,xj(k))$.
Here, we describe the possible improving of the nearest neighbour rule by the linear transformation (2) of the feature vectors xj(k):

$$yj(k) = A \ xj(k) \tag{12}$$

where A is [2 x n] matrix with the vectors w1 and w2 (2) as the two rows. As the result, the Euclidean distance functions $\delta y(y0,yj(k))$ (4) can be expressed as:

$$\delta y \ 2(y0,yj(k)) = (y0- yj(k))T(y0 - yj(k)) = (x0 - xj(k))TATA \ (x0 - xj(k)) \tag{13}$$

A quadratic matrix ATA can be represented in accordance with the spectral decomposition rule by their eigenvectors ki and eigenvalues $\chi i$ (ATA ki = $\chi i$ ki , $\| ki \| = <ki, ki >1/2 = 1$ ) [5]:

$$ATA = \chi 1 \ k1 \ k1T + \chi 2 \ k2 \ k2T \tag{14}$$

From the above:

$$\delta y \ 2(y0,yj(k)) = \chi 1 <k1, (x0- xj(k))>2 + \chi 2 <k2, (x0- xj(k))>2$$
$$= \delta x \ 2(x0,xj(k)) \ [\chi 1 \ cos2\alpha(k1, (x0- xj(k))) + \chi 2 \ cos2\alpha(k2, (x0- xj(k)))] \tag{15}$$

where $\alpha(ki, (x0- xj(k))$ is the angle between the eigenvector ki and the vector (x0- xj(k)).
As we can see from (15), the dependence of the distance $\delta y(y0,yj(k))$ between the transformed vectors y0 and yj(k) (12) on the distance $\delta x(x0,xj(k))$ between the feature vectors x0 and xj(k) can be modified by changing of the vectors w1 and w2 (2).

The ball $By(y0,K)$ (10) centred in the point $y0 = Ax0$ (12) and containing $K'$ ranked points $yj(k)$ (9) can be defined in a similar manner to (10) by using of the Euclidean distance $\delta y(y0,yj(i))$ (4):

$$By(y0,K) = \{yj(k): \delta y(y0,yj(i)) \leq \delta y(y0,yj(K'))\} \tag{16}$$

Let us assume that the symbol $Cx(x0,K')$ stands for a such set of $K'$ feature vectors $xj(k)$ from the ball $Bx(x0,K)$ (10), that are transformed by (12) into $By(y0,K')$ (16), where $K' < K$:

$$Cx(x0,K') = \{ xj(k): xj(k) \in Bx(x0,K) \text{ (10) and } yj(k) \in By(y0,K'), \text{ where } yj(k) \text{ is given by (12)}\} \tag{17}$$

The $K'$ nearest neighbours type of diagnosis support rule (10) can be based on the set $B'(x0)$ (17):

If the most of the labelled vectors $xj(k)$ from the set $Cx(x0,K')$ (17) belong to the disease $\omega k$, $\hspace{4cm}$ (18)
then the patient represented by $x0$ should be related to this disease.
We are proposing here a heuristic procedure aimed at optimisation of the rule (18) by a special choice of the vectors $w1$ and $w2$ in the transformation (2).

## 5. The Separability Postulates

In our approach, the choice of the vectors $w1$ and $w2$ (2) is done through minimisation of the differential criterion function $\Phi(w)$ (8) adjusting to the below separability postulate [4], [5]:

The linear transformation (12) should shorten the clear dipoles $\{xj(k), xj'(k)\}$ from the control set $Ic$ and lengthen the mixed dipoles $\{xj(k), x j'(k')\}$ belonging to the control set $Im$.
Let us pay the attention to the control sets $Ic$ and $Im$ containing such dipoles $\{xj(k), x j'(k')\}$, which are build from the elements $xj(k)$ and $x j'(k')$ belonging to the ball $Bx(x0,K)$ (10).
Let us consider at the beginning the linear transformation from the multidimensional space onto the line $y1 = <w1,x>$ (2). In this case, the separability postulate could be related to the following inequalities:

$$(\forall(j,j') \in Ic) - \beta c \; \delta x2(j,j') < <w1, x j(k) - x j'(k)> < \beta c \; \delta x2(j,j') \tag{19}$$

$$(\forall(j,j') \in Im+) <w1, xj(k) - x j'(k')> > \beta m \; \delta x2(j,j') \tag{20}$$

$$(\forall(j,j') \in Im-) <w1, xj(k) - xj'(k')> < -\beta m \; \delta x2(j,j') \tag{21}$$

where $\delta x2(j,j')$ (3) is the length of the dipole $\{xj(k), x\,j'(k')\}$, $\beta c$ is the shortening parameter ($0 \le \beta c \le 1$) and $\beta m$ is the lengthening parameter ($\beta m \ge 1$). Im+ and Im- are disjoined subsets of the control set Im (Im+ $\cup$ Im- = Im) of the mixed dipoles with the positive and negative orientation, adequately (Def. 2). Ic is the control set of the clear dipoles $\{xj(k), xj(k)\}$.

The penalty functions $\phi jj'+(w)$ (5) and $\phi jj'-(w)$ (6) can be adjusted to (19) by:

$$(\forall(j,j')) \in Ic)\ ajj' = \beta c\ \delta x2(j,j')\ and\ bjj' = -\beta c\ \delta x2(j,j') \tag{21}$$
$$and\ \ (\forall(j,j')) \in Im+)\ bjj' = \beta m\ \delta x2(j,j')\ and\ (\forall(j,j')) \in Im-)\ ajj' = -\beta m\ \delta x2(j,j')$$

We can remark, that such vector $w1^*$, which fulfils one of the inequalities (19) for the clear dipole $\{xj(k),xj'(k)\}$ decreases the penalty to zero ($\phi jj'+(w1^*) = 0$ and $\phi jj'-(w1^*) = 0$. Similarly, fulfilling of the inequality (19) for the mixed and positively oriented dipole $\{xj(k),xj'(k)\}$ decreases the penalty to zero ($\phi jj'+(w1^*) = 0$). The minimal value $\Phi(w1^*)$ (7) is zero if and only if all the inequalities (19), (20) and (21) are fulfilled.

The criterion function $\Phi(w)$ (7) can be adjusted in accordance with the separability postulate separately for each axis of the visualising plane. The optimal vector $w1^*$ defining the first axis can be found in the above described manner. The optimal vector $w2^*$ defining the second axis can be found by minimisation of the criterion function $\Phi(w)$ (7) defined on the projected vectors $zj(k)$ ($zj(k) \perp w1^*$) and adjusted to the separability postulate by the inequalities (19), (20), (21) with modified margins $\beta'm$ and $\beta'c$ ($\beta'm > \beta'c > 0$) [4].

The linear transformations (2) allow to obtain the nearest neighbours rule (18) based on the proximity ball $Cx(x0,K')$ (17) centred in the feature vector $x0$ of a new patient. The proximity ball $Cx(x0,K')$ (17) determines the neighbourhood of the vector $x0$. The shape of the ball $Cx(x0,K')$ depends on transformation parameters $w1$ and $w2$ (2), which are optimised in accordance with the minimum of the criterion function $\Phi(w)$ (8) and the separability postulate. The shape of the ball $Cx(x0,K')$ can be optimised locally by defining adequately subsets Ic and Im (8) of dipoles constituted only by the vectors $xj(k)$ from a neighbourhood of the point $x0$.

The subsets Ic and Im (8) can contain such clear and mixed dipoles $\{xj(k), xj'(k')\}$, which are built from the feature vectors $xj(k)$ belonging to the Euclidean ball $Bx(x0,K)$ (10). This ball is centred in the point $x0$ and contains K' labelled vectors $xj(k)$. The number K should be significantly larger than the number K' of the elements $xj(k)$ of the ball $Cx(x0,K')$ (17) used in the rule (18). Such choice of the subsets Ic and Im (8) allow to influence locally the shape of the ball $Cx(x0,K')$. In other words, the shape of the ball $Cx(x0,K')$ (17) determining the decision rule (18) could be tuned in accordance with local properties of the feature space.

## 6. Concluding Remarks

Local shaping of the ball $Cx(x0,K')$ (17) in the diagnosis support rule (18) results in the nearest neighbours classification rule with the similarity measure (distance function) changing over the feature space. Optimisation of the similarity measure based on the separability postulate can be seen as a generalisation of the Fishers linear discriminant criterion, which is aimed at a good separation of categories [2], [6].

The local tuning of the diagnosis support rule (18) allows to decrease the error rate and to improve the quality of this rule in comparison with the rules constant over the whole feature space. Such effect has been observed in the experiments with different diagnosis support rules of the computer system Hepar [3]. The visualising transformations of the data could not only give a new insight into a structure of a diagnostic problem, but also allow to improve of the diagnosis support rules.

# References

[1]. J. L. Kolodner: Case-based Reasoning, Morgan Kaufmann, San Mateo, CA 1993.

[2]. O. R. Duda, P. E. Hart: Pattern Classification, Sec.. Edition. J. Wiley, New York, 2001

[3]. L. Bobrowski, H. Wasyluk, Diagnosis supporting rules of the Hepar system, pp. 1309 - 1313 in: MEDINFO 2001, Eds: V. L. Petel, R. Rogers, R. Haux, IOS Press, Amsterdam 2001

[4]. L. Bobrowski, M. Topczewska: "Linear visualising transformations and convex, piecewise linear criterion functions", Bioc. and Biom. Eng., pp. 69 - 78, Vol. 22, Nr.1, 2002

[5]. L. Bobrowski: "Medical diagnosis support with data transformation and visualisation", pp. 108 - 114 in: Lecture Notes of the ICB Seminars: Statistics and Clinical Practice, ed. by L. Bobrowski, J. Doroszewski, N. Victor, June 2002, Warsaw

[6]. R. A. Johnson, D. W. Wichern: Applied Multivariate Statistical Analysis, Prentice-Hall, Inc., Englewood Cliffs, New York, 1991

[7]. L. Bobrowski: "Design of piecewise linear classifiers from formal neurons by some basis exchange, Pattern Recognition, 24(9), pp. 863-870, 1991

# Inductive Learning of Simple Diagnostic Scores

Martin Atzmueller, Joachim Baumeister, and Frank Puppe

University of Würzburg, 97074 Würzburg, Germany
Department of Computer Science
Phone: +49 931 888-6746, Fax: +49 931 888-6732
{atzmueller, baumeister, puppe}@informatik.uni-wuerzburg.de

**Abstract.** Knowledge acquisition and maintenance in medical domains with a large application domain ontology is a difficult task. To reduce knowledge elicitation costs, semi-automatic learning methods can be used to support the expert. We propose *diagnostic scores* as a promising approach and present a method for inductive learning of diagnostic scores. It can be be refined incrementally by applying different types of background knowledge. We give an evaluation of the presented approach with a real-world case base.

## 1   Introduction

Constructing and in particular maintaining a knowledge base in medical domains is a difficult task. If the degree of connectivity between findings and diagnoses is potentially high, then managing the sheer number of relations is a major problem. Pure automatic learning method are usually not good enough to reach a quality comparable to manually built knowledge bases. However, they can be used to support the expert. In such semi-automatic scenarios, understandability and interpretability of the learned models is of prime importance. Ideally, the learning method constructs knowledge in the same representation the human expert favors.

A rather wide spread formalism for medical decision making are diagnostic scores, e.g. [1, 2]. For inferring a concept, a limited number of features is used in a regular and simple to interpret manner, which can be applied even without a computer. In its simplest form, each feature - if observed in a case - individually contributes one point to an account (score), and if the score exceeds a threshold, the concept is established. Variations concern using several categories instead of one point, acquiring both negative and positive contributions, and utilizing several thresholds to express different degrees, e.g. to differentiate between "possible" and "probable" for inferring a concept.

In comparison to general rules, scores usually have no logical combinations in the precondition. Compared to Bayesian nets, scores have much simpler relations than the probability tables. Similar to both, they can be arranged hierarchically, i.e. a concept inferred with a score can be used to infer another concept. Of course, scores can be refined into both formalisms, but are quite expressable in itself. We therefore propose *diagnostic scores* as a promising approach to support knowledge engineering. Thus starting with automatically learned knowledge, the expert is able to use the learned knowledge as a starting point in constructing a knowledge base, such that the knowledge can be refined, tuned and extended as needed. One measure for the quality of a score

P. Perner et al. (Eds.): ISMDA 2003, LNCS 2868, pp. 23–30, 2003.

is the accuracy of inferring the respective concept. A second important criterion is the complexity of the score, e.g. depending on the number of features used for the score. We present an inductive method for learning diagnostic scores paying special attention to compromise between both criteria. The method can be refined incrementally using different types of background knowledge, which improve the learned scores.

Our implementation and evaluation is based on the knowledge-based documentation and consultation system for sonography SONOCONSULT (an advanced and isolated part of HEPATOCONSULT [3]) based on the diagnostic shell kit D3 [4]. This system is in routine use in the DRK-hospital in Berlin/Köpenick. The cases are detailed descriptions of findings of the examination(s), together with the inferred diagnoses (concepts). Both observations and diagnoses may be ordered hierarchically according to a specialization hierarchy from general to more detailed elements. This setting yields a high quality of the case base with detailed and usually correct case descriptions.

The rest of the paper is organized as follows: In Section 2 we introduce the basic notions, diagnostic scores and their basic properties. In Section 3 we first give essential basic definitions for the general learning task. Then we describe the method of learning diagnostic scores, and discuss which additional knowledge can be applied and its effect. An evaluation with a real-world case base is given in Section 4. We will conclude the paper in Section 5 with a discussion of the presented work, and we show promising directions for future work.

## 2   Basic Definition and Notions

In the following we define necessary notions that are considered for the learning task. The basic definitions for this task are the following:

We define $\Omega_Q$ to be the universe of of all questions available in the problem domain. In context of machine learning methods, questions are commonly called *attributes*. The type of a question $q \in \Omega_Q$ depends on the value range $dom(q)$. The value range can consist of numerical or symbolic values. A question $q \in \Omega_Q$ assigned to a value $v \in dom(q)$ is called a *finding* and we call $\Omega_{\mathcal{F}}$ the set of all possible findings in the given problem domain. A finding $f \in \Omega_{\mathcal{F}}$ is denoted by $q{:}v$ for $q \in \Omega_Q$ and $v \in dom(q)$.

Let $d$ be a *diagnosis* representing a possible solution and let $\Omega_{\mathcal{D}}$ be the universe of all possible diagnoses for a given problem domain. A diagnosis $d \in \Omega_{\mathcal{D}}$ is assigned to a symbolic state $dom(d) = \{excluded, unclear, probable\}$ with respect to a given problem. Let $\Omega_C$ be the universe of all possible cases. A case $c \in \Omega_C$ is defined as a tuple

$$c = (\mathcal{F}_c, \mathcal{D}_c, \mathcal{I}_c),$$

where $\mathcal{F}_c \in \Omega_{\mathcal{F}}$ is the set of findings observed in the case $c$. These findings are commonly called *problem description*. The set $\mathcal{D}_c \in \Omega_{\mathcal{D}}$ is the set of diagnoses describing the solution of the case, i.e. which habe been assigned to the state *probable*. The set $\mathcal{I}_c$ contains additional (meta-)information describing the case $c$ in more detail. For the learning task, we consider a case base $CB \subseteq \Omega_C$ containing all available cases that have been solved previously.

A simple and intuitive way for representing inferential knowledge is the utilization of *diagnostic scores* [5]. Then simple scoring rules are applied.

**Definition 1 (Simple Scoring Rule).** A *simple scoring rule* $r$ is denoted as follows:

$$r = f \xrightarrow{s} d,$$

where $f \in \Omega_{\mathcal{F}}$ and $d \in \Omega_{\mathcal{D}}$ is the targeted diagnosis. For each rule a symbolic confirmation category $s \in \Omega_{scr}$ is attached with $\Omega_{scr} \in \{ S_3, S_2, S_1, 0, S_{-1}, S_{-2}, S_{-3} \}$.

Let $\Omega_R$ be the universe of all possible rules for the sets $\Omega_{\mathcal{F}}$, $\Omega_{\mathcal{D}}$ and $\Omega_{scr}$. Then, we call $\mathcal{R} \subseteq \Omega_R$ the *rule base* containing the inferential knowledge of the problem domain.

Scores are used to represent a qualitative degree of uncertainty. In contrast to quantitative approaches, e.g. Bayesian methods, symbolic categories state the degree of confirmation or disconfirmation for diagnoses. In this way, a symbolic category $s$ expresses the uncertainty for which the observation of finding $f$ will confirm/disconfirm the diagnosis $d$. Whereas $s \in \{S_1, S_2, S_3\}$ stand for confirming symbolic categories in ascending order, the categories $s \in \{S_{-1}, S_{-2}, S_{-3}\}$ are ascending categories for disconfirming a diagnosis. A rule with category 0 has no effect on the diagnosis' state and therefore is usually omitted from the rule base. It is worth noticing, that the value range $\Omega_{scr}$ of the possible symbolic categories is not fixed. For a more detailed (or coarse) representation of confirmation the value range may be extended (or reduced).

For a given case $c \in \Omega_C$ the final state of each diagnosis $d \in \Omega_{\mathcal{D}}$ is determined by evaluating the available scoring rules $r \in \mathcal{R}$ targeting $d$. Thus rules $r = f \xrightarrow{s} d$ contained in $\mathcal{R}$ are activated, iff $f$ is observed in case $c$, i.e. $f \in \mathcal{F}_c$. The symbolic categories of the activated rules are aggregated by adding the categories in a way, so that four equal categories result in the next higher category (e.g. $S_1 + S_1 + S_1 + S_1 = S_2$) and so that two equal categories with opposite sign nullify (e.g. $S_1 + S_{-1} = 0$). For a more detailed or coarse definition of $\Omega_{scr}$ the aggregation rules may be adapted. A diagnosis is assumed to be *probable* (i.e. part of the final solution of the case), if the aggregated score is greater or equal than the symbolic category $S_3$.

Scoring rules have proven to be useful in large medical knowledge bases, e.g. in the INTERNIST/QMR project [6, 7]. For our own work with the shell-kit D3, scores have been proven to be successful in many (large) knowledge system projects, e.g. in a geo-ecological application [8] or in medical domains [3] and technical domains [5] using generalized scores. In context of the PIT system, Fronhöfer and Schramm [9] investigated the probabilistic aspects of scores. The LEXMED [10] project is a successful application developed with the PIT system.

## 3   Learning Diagnostic Scores

In the following we will first discuss diagnostic profiles utilized in the learning method. Then we will briefly discuss necessary data preprocessing steps for the learning task. After that we will outline the method for inductive learning of diagnostic scores from cases.

Diagnostic profiles describe a compact case representation for each diagnosis. For a diagnosis $d \in \Omega_{\mathcal{D}}$ a diagnostic profile $P_d = (\mathcal{F}_d, frec_{\mathcal{F}})$ contains the findings $\mathcal{F}_d \subset \Omega_{\mathcal{F}}$ that occur most frequently with the diagnosis (frequencies stored in $frec_{\mathcal{F}}$).

Learning diagnostic profiles entails, that each profile will initially contain all findings which occur together with the profile's diagnoses. After that we apply a statistical pruning method, such that the profiles contain typical attributes and findings for a given diagnosis. For a more detailled discussion we refer to [11].

The basic algorithm for learning diagnostic scores can only handle discrete valued attributes. Therefore, for handling continuous data we will transform continuous attributes into attributes with discrete partitions in a preprocessing step. For some continuous attributes the expert already defined reasonable partitions. In the case, that there are predefined partitions available, we use these. Otherwise, we used a *k-means* clustering method for discretizing attribute values.

For learning diagnostic scores we first have to identify dependencies between findings and diagnoses. In general, all possible combinations between diagnoses and findings have to be taken into account. However, to reduce the search space, we first learn diagnostic profiles identifying typical findings for a diagnosis. In this way we restrict the set of *important* findings for a diagnosis using diagnostic profiles.

In summary, we basically apply four steps for learning a diagnostic scoring rule: we first identify a dependency association between a finding $f \in \Omega_{\mathcal{F}}$ and diagnosis $d \in \Omega_{\mathcal{D}}$, rate this dependency, map it to a symbolic category $s \in \Omega_{scr}$ and finally construct a diagnostic rule: $f \xrightarrow{s} d$.

---

**Algorithm 1** Learning Simple Diagnostic Scores

---

**Require:** Case base $CB \in \Omega_C$

1: **for all** diagnoses $d \in \Omega_{\mathcal{D}}$ **do**
2:     learn a diagnostic profile $P_d = (\mathcal{F}_d, frec_{\mathcal{F}})$
3:     **for all** attributes $q \in \{q \mid q \in \Omega_Q, \exists f \in dom(q), f \in \mathcal{F}_d)\}$ **do**
4:         **for all** findings $f \in dom(q)$ **do**
5:             construct binary variables $D, F$ for $d$ and $f$, which measure if $d$ and $f$ occur in cases of the case base $CB$.
6:             compute $\chi_{fd}^2 = \chi^2(F, D)$
7:             **if** $\chi_{fd}^2 >= \chi_\alpha^2$ **then**
8:                 compute the correlation/$\phi_{fd}$ coefficient $\phi_{fd} = \phi(F, D)$
9:                 **if** $\phi_{fd} >= treshold_c$ **then**
10:                    compute the quasi-probabilistic score $qps$,
                       $qps = sgn(\phi_{fd}) * prec(r)(1 - FAR(r))$ using the pseudo-rule: $f \rightarrow d$
11:                    map the $qps$-score to a symbolic category $s$ using a conversion table
12:                    if available, apply background knowledge to validate the diagnostic scoring rule
13:                    create a diagnostic scoring rule (if valid): $f \xrightarrow{s} d$

---

For each diagnosis $d$, we create a diagnostic profile. We consider all attributes (questions) in the profile selecting the findings which are observed in the case base. Then we create a four-fold contingency-table for each finding – diagnosis relation. With the given diagnosis $d$ and finding $f$ of attribute $q$, i.e. $f = q{:}v$, we construct two binary variables limiting these to cases $\mathcal{C} \subseteq CB$ from the case base in which attribute $q$ is not unknown: a variable $D$ which is true, iff diagnosis $d$ occurs in a case, and false otherwise, and a variable $F$ which is true, iff finding $f$ occurs in a case, otherwise $F$ is false likewise. We fill the four-fold table as shown below.

|            | $D = true$ | $D = false$ |
|------------|------------|-------------|
| $F = true$  | a          | b           |
| $F = false$ | c          | d           |

The frequency counts denoted in the table are defined as follows:

$$a = N(D = true \wedge F = true), \ b = N(D = false \wedge F = true),$$
$$c = N(D = true \wedge F = false), \ d = N(D = false \wedge F = false),$$

where $N(cond)$ is the number of times the condition $cond$ is true for cases $c \in C$. To identify dependencies between findings and diagnoses, we apply the $\chi^2$-*test for independence* with a certain threshold $\chi^2_\alpha$ corresponding to confidence level $\alpha$. For binary variables the formula for the $\chi^2$-test simplifies to

$$\chi^2(F, D) = \frac{(a + b + c + d)(ad - bc)^2}{(a + b)(c + d)(a + c)(b + d)}. \tag{1}$$

For small sample sizes, we apply the Yates' correction for a more accurate result. For all dependent tuples $(F, D)$ we derive the quality of the dependency using the $\phi$-coefficient

$$\phi(F, D) = \frac{ad - bc}{\sqrt{(a + b)(c + d)(a + c)(b + d)}}, \tag{2}$$

which measures the degree of association between two binary variables. We use it to discover positive or negative dependencies. If the absolute value of $\phi(F, D)$ is less than a certain threshold $threshold_c$, i.e. $|\phi(F, D)| < threshold_c$, then we do not consider this weak dependency for rule generation. For the remaining dependencies we generate rules described as follows: If $\phi(F, D) < 0$, then we obtain a negative association between the two variables, and we will generate a rule $f \xrightarrow{s} d$ with a negative category $s$. If $\phi(F, D) > 0$, then we construct a rule $f \xrightarrow{s} d$ with a positive category $s$.

For determining the exact symbolic confirmation category of the remaining rules $r = f \rightarrow d$, we utilize two measures used in diagnosis: *precision* and the *false alarm rate (FAR)*, which is also known as the *false positive rate*, or $1 -$ specificity. Precision is defined as $prec(r) = \frac{TP}{TP+FP}$, whereas the false alarm rate is defined as $FAR(r) = \frac{FP}{FP+TN}$. $TP, TN, FP$ denote the number of *true positives*, *true negatives*, and *false positives*, respectively. These can easily be extracted from the contingency table. For a positive dependency between finding $f$ and $d$, $TP = a$, $TN = d$ and $FP = b$. For a negative dependency the situation is different, since we try to predict the absence of the diagnosis, so $TP = b$, $TN = c$ and $FP = a$. To score the dependency, we first compute a *quasi probabilistic score (qps)* which we then map to a symbolic category. The numeric *qps* score is computed as follows:

$$qps(r) = sgn(\phi(D, F)) * prec(r)(1 - FAR(r)) \tag{3}$$

We achieve a tradeoff between the accuracy of the diagnostic scoring rule to predict a disease measured against all predictions and the proportion of false predictions. It is worth noting, that often the *true positive rate (TPr)* (which is also known as *recall/sensitivity*) is used in combination with the FAR as a measure of accuracy. However, this is mostly applicable to standard rules, which are more complex than diagnostic scores. Since a diagnostic score is a combination of several diagnostic scoring rules, which support each other in establishing a diagnosis, their accuracy needs to be assessed on localized regions of the diagnosis space. So, precision is more suggestive, since it does not take the complete diagnosis space into account, but it measures only the accuracy of the localized prediction. To ease interpretability of the discovered knowledge, we restrict the mapping process to only six different symbolic confirmation categories, three positive and three negative. The *qps*-scores are mapped to the symbolic categories according to the following conversion table:

| qps(r) | category(r) | qps(r) | category(r) |
|--------|-------------|--------|-------------|
| $[-1.0, -0.9]$ | $\rightharpoonup S_{-3}$ | $(0.0, 0.5)$ | $\rightharpoonup S_1$ |
| $[-0.9, -0.5]$ | $\rightharpoonup S_{-2}$ | $[0.5, 0.9)$ | $\rightharpoonup S_2$ |
| $[-0.5, 0.0)$ | $\rightharpoonup S_{-1}$ | $[0.9, 1.0]$ | $\rightharpoonup S_3$ |

We accept the loss of information to facilitate a user-friendly adaptation of the learned diagnostic scores by the expert in a later step.

*Including Background Knowledge* Sometimes *abnormality* information about attribute values may be available. We will use these abnormalities, for further shrinking the size of the generated rule base: Let $r = q{:}v \xrightarrow{s} d$ be a given scoring rule. If $s \in \Omega_{scr}$ denotes a positive category and $v$ is a normal value of attribute $q$, then we will omit rule $r$, since findings describing normal behavior usually should not increase the confirmation of a diagnosis. Furthermore, if $s$ denotes a negative category and $v$ is an abnormal value of attribute $q$, then we likewise will omit rule $r$, because an abnormal finding usually should not decrease the confirmation of a diagnosis.

As a second type of background knowledge the expert can provide *partition class* knowledge describing how to divide the set of diagnoses and attributes into partially disjunctive subsets, i.e. partitions. These subsets correspond to certain problem areas of the application domain. For example, in the medical domain of sonography, we have subsets corresponding to problem areas like *liver, pancreas, kidney, stomach* and *intestine*. This knowledge is especially useful when diagnosing multiple faults. Since a case may contain multiple solutions, attributes occurring with several diagnoses will be contained in several diagnostic profiles. To give additional support to the dependencies which are discovered, for each such dependency $f \rightarrow d$ we check, if attribute $q$ with $f = q{:}v$ and diagnosis $d$ are in the same partition class. If the check fails, then we prune the dependency, which reduces noise and irrelevant dependencies.

*Diagnostic Scoring Rule Post-Processing* To reduce the number of generated rules, and to make them more comprehensible, we merge rules for continuous attributes. We combine rules covering neighboring partitions of attributes into one rule, if they have equal symbolic categories. This does not result in a loss of accuracy, because the rule base is not changed semantically, but only tightened syntactically.

## 4   Evaluation

We evaluated the presented methods with cases taken from a medical application, which is currently in routine use. The applied SONOCONSULT case base contains 1340 cases, with a mean of diagnoses $M_d = 4.32 \pm 2.79$ and a mean of relevant findings $M_f = 76.89 \pm 20.59$ per case.

For the evaluation of our experiments we adopted the commonly used F-measure known from information extraction theory which is appropriate for comparing solutions with multiple faults. For the correct solution $\mathcal{D}_1$ and an inferred solution $\mathcal{D}_2$ the F-measure is defined as follows $(\mathcal{D}_1, \mathcal{D}_2 \subseteq \Omega_\mathcal{D})$:

$$f(\mathcal{D}_1, \mathcal{D}_2) = \frac{(\beta^2 + 1) \cdot prec(\mathcal{D}_1, \mathcal{D}_2) \cdot recall(\mathcal{D}_1, \mathcal{D}_2)}{\beta^2 \cdot prec(\mathcal{D}_1, \mathcal{D}_2) + recall(\mathcal{D}_1, \mathcal{D}_2)} , \qquad (4)$$

where $\beta$ denotes a constant weight for the precision and $prec(\mathcal{D}_1, \mathcal{D}_2) = |\mathcal{D}_1 \cap \mathcal{D}_2|/|\mathcal{D}_2|$, $recall(\mathcal{D}_1, \mathcal{D}_2) = |\mathcal{D}_1 \cap \mathcal{D}_2|/|\mathcal{D}_1|$. We used $\beta = 1$ for our experiments.

For the evaluation we applied a stratified 10-fold cross-validation method. We applied two different settings for learning scores, first using no background knowledge for the learning task (-K) and secondly applying all available background knowledge (+K), i.e. abnormality and partition class knowledge. We created several sets of scores depending on the parameter $threshold_c$. Two criteria, accuracy and complexity of the learned scores, were used for assessing the quality of the scores. A score is considered to be the more complex, the more findings it contains. This directly corresponds to the number of learned rules per diagnosis (rules/d Mean, with a standard deviation rules/d SD). An overall impression of the complexity of the learned scores is given by the total number of learned rules (rules). Furthermore, as a global complexity measure we count the number of findings/questions which are used in the learning process. Usually a moderate number of findings/questions is considered more comprehensible than a huge number of findings/questions. The results are presented in the following table.

| $threshold_c$ | rules | | rules/d Mean | | rules/d SD | | questions | | findings | | accuracy | |
|---|---|---|---|---|---|---|---|---|---|---|---|---|
| | -K | +K | -K | +K | -K | +K | -K | +K | -K | +K | -K | +K |
| 0.10 | 3867 | 956 | 53.71 | 13.27 | 29.54 | 8.43 | 135 | 91 | 403 | 224 | 0.96 | 0.91 |
| 0.20 | 2494 | 673 | 34.64 | 9.34 | 19.78 | 5.88 | 135 | 88 | 393 | 193 | 0.96 | 0.90 |
| 0.30 | 1692 | 484 | 23.50 | 6.73 | 12.66 | 3.80 | 132 | 83 | 357 | 164 | 0.94 | 0.89 |
| 0.40 | 1213 | 364 | 16.85 | 5.06 | 8.72 | 2.49 | 126 | 77 | 307 | 143 | 0.92 | 0.87 |
| 0.50 | 890 | 272 | 12.36 | 3.77 | 6.43 | 1.68 | 118 | 72 | 264 | 124 | 0.91 | 0.87 |
| 0.60 | 674 | 212 | 9.36 | 2.94 | 4.49 | 1.23 | 111 | 66 | 226 | 110 | 0.86 | 0.81 |

The high values for the accuracy for low values of $threshold_c$ and the large number of rules per diagnosis indicate overfitting of the learned knowledge. This is of course domain dependent, and therefore the expert needs to tune the threshold carefully. With greater values for $threshold_c$ less rules are generated, since only strong dependencies are taken into account. If $threshold_c$ is too high, i.e. if too many rules are pruned, this obviously degrades the accuracy of the learned scores. Applying background knowledge has clearly the effect of strongly reducing the number of scoring rules which are learned, by removing irrelevant and noisy findings from the scoring rules, and thus pruning the scores effectively. Thus, a set of scores with moderate complexity can be obtained, which still yield a sufficient accuracy level.

## 5  Conclusion

We presented a method for learning simple scoring rules applied for diagnostic tasks. Scoring rules are appealing because of their simplicity and practical relevance in medical decision making. The presented work investigates methods for learning small and simple sets of rules with an acceptable quality concerning diagnostic accuracy and rule complexity. Background knowledge, like abnormalities for attribute values further helped to shrink the size of the rule base, without significantly reducing the accuracy. The evaluation of our methods was implemented using a stratified 10-cross validation applying 1340 cases from a real-life medical application.

In the future, we are planning to improve the presented work by considering subgroups for score extraction, which can focus the scores on significant subspaces of the diagnoses' space. Furthermore, scores can be refined and simplified by aggregating findings into sub-concepts by learning sub-scores first, and using these sub-scores in combination with other findings for the final scores. Another promising approach is the automatic adaptation of thresholds for scores. We expect such ideas to be a good start for significantly improving the combination of accuracy and complexity of the scores.

## References

[1] Ohmann, C., et al.: Clinical Benefit of a Diagnostic Score for Appendicitis: Results of a Prospective Interventional Study. Archives of Surgery **134** (1999) 993–996

[2] Eich, H.P., Ohmann, C.: Internet-Based Decision-Support Server for Acute Abdominal Pain. Artificial Intelligence in Medicine **20** (2000) 23–36

[3] Buscher, H.P., Engler, C., Fuhrer, A., Kirschke, S., Puppe., F.: HepatoConsult: A Knowledge-Based Second Opinion and Documentation System. Artificial Intelligence in Medicine **24** (2002) 205–216

[4] Puppe, F.: Knowledge Reuse Among Diagnostic Problem-Solving Methods in the Shell-Kit D3. Int. J. Human-Computer Studies **49** (1998) 627–649

[5] Puppe, F., Ziegler, S., Martin, U., Hupp, J.: Wissensbasierte Diagnosesysteme im Service-Support. Springer Verlag (2001)

[6] R., M., Pople, H.E., Myers, J.: Internist-1, an Experimental Computer-Based Diagnostic Consultant for General Internal Medicine. NEJM **307** (1982) 468–476

[7] Pople, H.E.: Heuristic Methods for Imposing Structure on Ill-Structured Problems: The Structuring of Medical Diagnostics. In Szolovits, P., ed.: Artificial Intelligence in Medicine. AAAS, Westview Press (1982)

[8] Neumann, M., Baumeister, J., Liess, M., Schulz, R.: An Expert System to Estimate the Pesticide Contamination of Small Streams using Benthic Macroinvertebrates as Bioindicators, Part 2. Ecological Indicators **2** (2003) 391–401

[9] Fronhöfer, B., Schramm, M.: A Probability Theoretic Analysis of Score Systems. In Kern-Isberner, G., Lukasiewicz, T., Weydert, E., eds.: KI-2001 Workshop: Uncertainty in Artificial Intelligence. (2001) 95–108

[10] Schramm, M., Ertel, W.: Reasoning with Probabilities and Maximum Entropy: The System PIT and its Application in LEXMED. In et al., K.I., ed.: Operations Research Proceeedings, Springer Verlag (1999) 274–280

[11] Baumeister, J., Atzmueller, M., Puppe, F.: Inductive Learning for Case-Based Diagnosis with Multiple Faults. In: Advances in Case-Based Reasoning. Volume 2416 of LNAI. Springer-Verlag, Berlin (2002) 28–42 Proceedings of the 6th European Conference on Case-Based Reasoning (ECCBR-2002).

# A Virtual Approach to Integrating Biomedical Databases and Terminologies

V. Maojo[1], M. García-Remesal[2], H. Billhardt[1],
J. Crespo[3], F. Martín-Sánchez[4], A. Sousa-Pereira[1]

[1]Biomedical Informatics Group, Polytechnical University of Madrid, SPAIN
[2]Artificial Intelligence Group, University King Juan Carlos, Madrid, SPAIN
[3] Bioinformatics Unit (BIOTIC), Institute of Health Carlos III, Madrid, SPAIN
[4] University of Aveiro/IEETA, PORTUGAL
vmaojo@fi.upm.es

**Abstract:** INFOGENMED is an informatics and telematics project, funded by the IST directorate of the European Commission. In this paper, we present our current achievements and plans to develop a series of tools to provide on-line integration of remote medical and genetic databases through a common, Web-based browser. Users at research and professional settings will soon need guided access to a wide range of medical (e.g, clinical databases, medical records) and biological (e.g., genomic and proteomic databases) sources. Most of this information is currently located at different heterogeneous databases and data warehouses, including diverse schemas, vocabularies, query languages and restricted access. We have chosen a virtual repository approach for the project. We briefly describe an unification approach to integrate the contents of the databases. By using this kind of projects, users can access different remote sources and retrieve the information they are looking for. Once this information is available, different data analysis methods (such as data mining techniques) can be used in order to extract patterns and knowledge.

## 1. Introduction

The completion of the human and other genome projects and the development of bioinformatics methods and tools in biomedical research and care promise to introduce novel medical applications of genetic information, including diagnostic and therapeutic procedures. From this vision, medical informatics and bioinformatics researchers need new informatics tools are needed to achieve an optimal integration of genetic and clinical information, which are currently available at remote sites.

Biomedical professionals currently need new approaches for collaborative research efforts that may lead to new directions in genomic medicine. Research in the biomedical sciences has generated a great deal of genetic information located at different world sites that health professionals may use to create novel diagnostic and therapeutic procedures in medicine. Therefore, physicians will need new methods and tools to

P. Perner et al. (Eds.): ISMDA 2003, LNCS 2868, pp. 31–38, 2003.

access, search, and retrieve useful information from distributed and heterogeneous biomedical sources.

The integration of distributed, heterogeneous biomedical data sources present research challenges, such as: i) Information has to be located, accessed, and retrieved from different sites over the Internet, and ii) Data exchange is difficult since biomedical data sources may present different formats, coding, and terminologies [1].

Biomedical terminologies will be a key component of future integrated information systems. To share and reuse these terminologies, it will be necessary a conceptual integration of terms from different vocabularies. Vocabulary servers are needed to achieve such conceptual integration and also to assist in the integration of heterogeneous information sources — e.g. to resolve semantic incompatibilities — or to enhance searches [2].

## 2. Objectives and Desired Functionality of the INFOGENMED Project

The main objectives of the INFOGENMED project [3] are: i) to facilitate the identification, access, integration, and retrieval of genetic and medical information from heterogeneous databases over Internet, through virtual repositories and ii) to develop a research direction for the exchange and unification of medical and genetic terminologies, stored in vocabulary servers.

Users can access the INFOGENMED system via a conventional web browser. Once they are connected to the system, they can query different virtual repositories through an unified and user-friendly interface. This will provide a protocol-based "wizard" to explain users how to use the INFOGENMED system to carry out a scientific research, according to their personal profile — e.g., physician, molecular biologist, epidemiologist, etc.— and the kind of information they want to access.

A virtual repository is an information resource that does not physically exist, but gives users the perception of working with a single local repository that integrates data from one or more information sources [4]. A virtual repository may encapsulate either an actual, physical database — e.g. public web databases such as MEDLINE, GENBANK, or OMIM or other private medical and genetic databases located at different biomedical research centers — or a set of pre-existing virtual repositories. The objective of INFOGENMED is to integrate the information contents of all them.

The vocabulary server can also be queried by users to get information, such as definitions of concepts, synonyms, codes corresponding to different codification schemas for a given term, etc. The vocabulary server may also be used to enhance searches — e.g., to make searches using standard terminologies or to include synonyms in the search process to avoid losing relevant information.

## 3. Proposed Architecture for the INFOGENMED Project

In this section, the proposed architecture for the INFOGENMED project is described. Figure 1, adapted from a previous report [5], shows a general overview of the project in its current state. External users from different hospitals or research centers can access different databases located over Internet — in the picture, these databases are called "external databases" — that include both public web databases and other private biomedical databases located at different remote sites. All these databases are maintained and curated by their owners at their respective institutions, keeping data updated. Databases marked as "internal databases" — and that are protected behind a firewall — are maintained by members of the INFOGENMED consortium. In the context of the project, we plan to include a database of rare genetic diseases, created and maintained by members of the Institute of Health Carlos III from Madrid (Spain).

"Internal users" are members of the INFOGENMED consortium that are authorized to update internal databases and to administrate the INFOGENMED system. The administration of the INFOGENMED system includes tasks such as adding new data sources to the system, creating new virtual repositories, and other administrative issues.

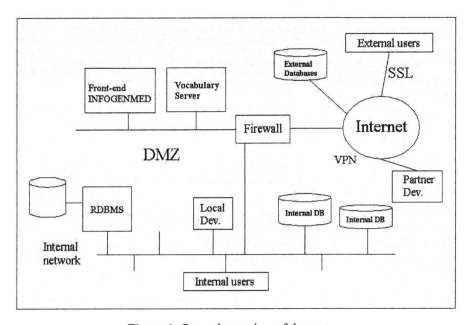

**Figure 1.** General overview of the system.

The user interface module provides users with access to the INFOGENMED system. External users can query the available virtual repositories via a user-friendly query interface. It also provides functionalities to query the vocabulary server, through the terminology browser, to obtain definitions of concepts, terms related to a given term, synonyms, etc., using this information to enhance searches. As stated above, the protocol-based assistant can be used to help users in managing the INFOGENMED system. This module provides internal users various facilities and tools to administrate the services provided by the database integration engine module.

This module also allows internal users to create new virtual repositories by translating the physical schema of a real database into a conceptual schema. This translation is achieved using a mapping facility. This mapping facility allows internal users to map entities, attributes, and relationships from the physical schema of the real database into semantically similar concepts, relationships, and attributes that may be obtained via the terminology server. Note that this translation requires user interaction to resolve semantic incompatibilities, so it cannot be performed automatically. At this moment, we are considering the possibility of using an ontology-based representation for the conceptual schemas of virtual repositories.

This module also allows to integrate the information space of two or more pre-existing virtual repositories that belong to the same or related domains, by means of the unification engine. This step can be performed automatically via an unification algorithm, as described in [3].

Once results have been returned by the different databases affected by the query, they must be integrated, formatted, and then presented to the user. Some data sources, and more concretely, some public web databases such as MEDLINE return their results embedded into an HTML page. In these cases, it is necessary to "extract" the relevant information from the HTML page and perform the inverse mapping between this information and the concepts, relationships, or attributes that belong to its conceptual schema, which is stored within its corresponding virtual repository.

## 4. A Virtual Repository Approach

As stated above, the INFOGENMED project has adopted virtual repositories as the technological and conceptual approach to integrate distributed and heterogeneous databases. Following this approach, to connect a new database to INFOGENMED, we have to translate its physical schema into a common conceptual representation that we have called "the virtual repository conceptual schema". This translation is carried out by mapping entities, attributes, and relationships from the physical database schema to "standard" concepts, attributes, and relationships supplied by a terminology server. Note that this translation requires user interaction to be performed.

Queries launched to the INFOGENMED system necessarily have to be written in the INFOGENMED query language — IQL from now onwards. This query language has to meet the following requirements: (1) It must be a declarative language — i.e. users have to specify what do they want, but they do not have to indicate how to get it. (2) It must provide users to access the whole information space corresponding to a virtual repository — i.e. every entity, attribute, or relationship belonging to its conceptual schema. (3) It must translate queries issued to the conceptual schema of a given virtual repository into queries for its children's conceptual schemas. When the lowest level of the hierarchy — i.e. real databases — has been reached, it must translate conceptual queries, expressed in IQL, into queries expressed in the native query language supported by each real data source. (4) It must allow users to perform operations similar to those from relational algebra: selection, projection, union, etc.

In summary, the IQL query language has to be general and expressive enough to query the conceptual model of virtual repositories. At the current state we are exploring how to conceptualize the space of information of virtual repositories. Ontologies may be an adequate option.

## 5. Integrating and Accessing Medical and Genetic Terminologies

Medical Informatics researchers have dedicated considerable efforts during the last decades to create unified medical terminologies and coding [2]. For instance, the Unified Medical Language System (UMLS) and the MeSH terms, used in various applications (e.g., to classify and optimise bibliographic searches in MEDLINE), have been created at the US National Library of Medicine (NLM). Later, some informatics systems were created to manage and use these vocabularies in various applications.

Similarly, an increasing interest has appeared in the last years in Bioinformatics regarding genetic terminology — e.g. Gene ontology [6], Human Gene Nomenclature. Some genetic terms are included in the UMLS and it is possible to carry out bibliographic searches in MEDLINE to retrieve papers related to genomics or genetics. Nevertheless, there is not an unified method to access and retrieve integrated medical and genetic information from remote databases from a clinical perspective.

One of the future objectives of INFOGENMED is to use an integrated ontology in the project, linking concepts from medicine and biology. At this moment, there are no integrated biomedical ontologies providing the kind of functionalities that we need for the project, although some kind of integration (e.g., UMLS-gene ontology) is expected shortly.

## 6. User Interface. Protocols

In the INFOGENMED project one of the objectives is to provide biomedical practitioners with tools to guide research and clinical routine. In the context of biomedical settings, with technologies such as microarrays and other diagnostic and management genetic tools, some kind of training and guidance will be needed to use genomic information in patient care.

We have created different kinds of tools to store protocol-based guidance for clinicians and biologists in terms of using clinical, genomic and genetic data and information. Since various databases and information sources are already available over Internet and other federated databases can be integrated in a project such as IN-FOGENMED, the system might also provide clear indications to non-informatics users about where the information needed is located and how can be accessed and retrieved. This kind of information is not too different from the kind of information that is currently available in various representations of clinical practice guidelines and protocols, in paper or computer-based formats [7].

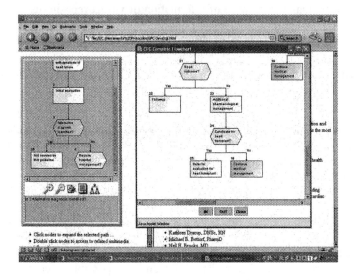

**Figure 2.** A flowchart-based representation of user-centered protocols for accessing information, adapted from [8].

Clinical practice guidelines and protocols have been traditionally represented, stored, disseminated and used in paper format. Over the last years, different institutions have realized the advantages that computer implementations of protocols can give to professionals and users.

A flowchart shows the logical steps designed to manage each clinical situation. All nodes include information that will appear in the graphical representation and can be linked to related multimedia information and external sources of information. For instance, a node may indicate to connect a database such as OMIM or MEDLINE. The description of dependencies among nodes determines the structure of the flow-chart.

Remote users can visualize algorithms graphically, accessing multimedia information related to each clinical problem. Since protocols can be viewed using any WWW browser with Java compliance, the system can be used by people with low training in computers.

Java tools and technologies facilitate platform-independent access and display of multimedia information. An important reason for local adaptation is variability in medical practice. For instance, a specific genetic test or recommendation cannot be carried out at some medical centers. The guideline can be adapted to their specific clinical environments and circumstances, including different kinds of biological and medical informations.

## 7. Conclusions and Future Directions

The INFOGENMED project is an integrated approach for sharing and exchanging medical and genetic information. In our vision, we expect that systems like this could facilitate biomedical reseachers the methods and tools needed to create virtual laboratories.

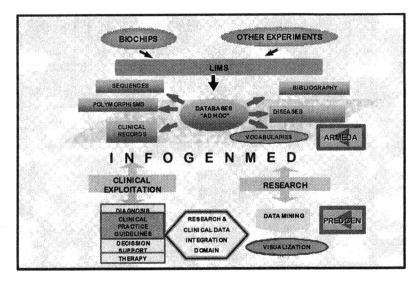

**Figure 3.** A proposal for future uses of INFOGENMED

In these Internet-based environments users will access and manage a significant part of the information they need using their computers. While efforts for integrating heterogenous databases have been developed for more than a decade [9, 10,11,12], new research approaches for integrating medical and biological sources and terminologies face new challenges, as it has been explained in this paper.

## Acknowledgements

Part of this project has been funded by the European Commission (IST INFOGEN-MED project), the Spanish Ministry of Health (INBIOMED network), and the Spanish Ministry of Science and Technology (MEDGENBASE).

# References

1. Sujansky, W: "Heterogeneous Database Integration in Biomedicine". Journal of Biomedical Informatics Vol. 34, No. 4, pp. 285-298 (2001).
2. Cimino, J.: Coding systems in healthcare. Methods of information in medicine, 35, pp. 273-284. 1996.
3. "INFOGENMED: A virtual laboratory for accessing and integrating genetic and medical information for health applications". EC Project IST-2001-39013. 2002-04.
4. Billhardt, H., Crespo, J., Maojo, V., Martin, F., Maté, JL.: "A New Method for Unifying Heterogeneous Databases". Proceedings of ISMDA 2001: 54-61.
5. García-Remesal, M., Crespo, J., Silva, A., Billhardt, H., Martín, F., Rodríguez-Pedrosa, J., Martín, V., Sousa, A., Babic, A., and Maojo, V.: "INFOGENMED: Integrating heterogeneous medical and genetic databases and terminologies". In: Proceedings of KES'2002. Crema (italy). September 2002.
6. The Gene Ontology Consortium: "Gene Ontology: tool for the unification of biology". Nature Genetics, Vol. 25, pp. 25-29 (2000).
7. Society for Medical Decision Making Committee of Standardization of Clinical Algorithms. Proposal for Clinical Algorithm Standards. Medical Decision Making. 1992; 12(2): 149-154.
8. Maojo, V.; Herrero, C.; Valenzuela, F.; Crespo J, Lázaro P., and Pazos, A. A Java based multimedia tool for clinical practice guidelines. Proceedings of medical informatics europe 1997. Porto carras, Greece.
9. Wiederhold, G.: "Mediators in the Architecture of Future Information Systems". IEEE Computer, Vol. 25, No. 3, pp. 38-49 (1992).
10. Gruber, T.: "A translation approach to portable ontology specifications". Knowledge Acquisition, Vol. 5, No. 2, pp. 199-220 (1993).
11. Y. Arens, C.Y. Chee, C.N. Hsu, C.A. Knoblock: "Retrieving and integrating data from multiple information sources". International Journal of Intelligent and Cooperative Information Systems, No. 2, Vol. 2, pp. 127-158 (1993).
12. Baker, P., Brass, A., Bechhofer, S., Goble, C., Paton, N., Stevens, R. "TAMBIS: Transparent Access to Multiple Bioinformatics Information Sources. An Overview". Proceedings of the Sixth International Conference on Intelligent Systems for Molecular Biology, ISMB98, Montreal, 1998.

# Data Mining with Meva in MEDLINE

Holger Tenner[1], Gerda Roswitha Thurmayr[2], Rudolf Thurmayr[2]

Institut für Medizinische Statistik und Epidemiologie
Klinikum rechts der Isar, TU München (IMSE)
Ismaninger Str. 22, 81675 München
[1] http://www.med-ai.com/
[2] http://www.imse.med.tu-muenchen.de/

**Abstract.** A simple search with PubMed in MEDLINE, the world's largest medical database, results quite often in a listing of many articles with little relevance for the user. Therefore a medico-scientific data mining web service called Meva (MEDLINE Evaluator) was developed, capable of analyzing the bibliographic fields returned by an inquiry to PubMed. Meva converts these data into a well-structured expressive result, showing a graphical condensed representation of counts and relations of the fields using histograms, correlation tables, detailed sorted lists or MeSH trees. The user can specify filters or minimal frequencies to restrict the analysis in the data mining process. MeSH codes for MeSH terms may be listed. Furthermore he can limit the output on first authors. Results can be delivered as HTML or in a delimited format to import into any database.

## 1   Introduction

Medical on-line databases are getting more and more popular. According to a market study (API study 2001, published by "LA-MED Kommunikationsforschung im Gesundheitswesen"), 37.2% of general practitioners and practicing internists younger than 40 years in Germany use medical on-line databases like MEDLINE.

If the user chooses MEDLINE as data source, a good recall for his retrieval is ensured: MEDLINE is the largest medical database; most of the important medical journals are included in MEDLINE.

If the user chooses PubMed as distribution platform for MEDLINE, he will get these data free of charge and without the need of installing additional retrieval software – any web browser will do it. Other distributions like OVID or WinSPIRS are provided with costs and additional retrieval software.

Nevertheless, a simple search in MEDLINE with PubMed results quite often in dozens of articles with more or less little precision for the user. Besides, PubMed displays the result as an unstructured list. The client is free to sort this list for authors, journals or publication dates, but there is no possibility to condense these data.

For that reason, an interactive data mining web service called *Meva* was developed to concentrate and display PubMed's results in a more graphical way. With *data mining*, a not-trivial and automated search for knowledge in mass data is denoted [3].

P. Perner et al. (Eds.): ISMDA 2003, LNCS 2868, pp. 39–46, 2003.

## 2   Meva

*Meva* (*MEDLINE evaluator*) is a free medico-scientific data mining web service hosted at http://www.med-ai.com/ and at the intranet of IMSE, TU München.

Unlike many PubMed web portals, it works as a PubMed postprocessor: it analyses the result returned by an inquiry to PubMed which has to be saved to a file for this purpose. Meva converts the information of a PubMed retrieval outcome into a well-structured expressive result, showing a graphical condensed representation of counts and relations of the bibliographic fields.

### 2.1   Operational Architecture of Meva and Related Systems

The user searches in MEDLINE with PubMed and saves the result to a file on his computer. Afterwards, he consults Meva via its web consultation form (Fig. 1).

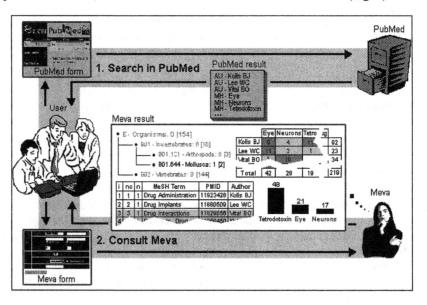

**Fig. 1.** Operational architecture of Meva

### 2.2   Meva's Input

Meva is controlled by its associated web form, the Meva consultation form. The user interface is available in English and German. An example shall illustrate the usage.

In this example, the user searched with the expression *Optical illusion[mh] 2000[dp]* in PubMed for articles indexed with the MeSH term *Optical illusions* and published in 2000. He saved his result as MEDLINE format to the file *Optical_illusion[mh]_2000[dp].txt* on his computer.

In Meva's consultation form, he selected the bibliographic field *MeSH terms* as the first and *Author* as the second interesting field, the path to the saved PubMed file and some other parameters which are explained below (Fig. 2).

## Consult Meva about your PubMed data

| Parameter | | Field 1 | Field 2 |
|---|---|---|---|
| | Bibliogr. field | MeSH Terms ▾ | Author ▾ |
| Input | Search filter | * <br> ☐ Ignore case <br> ☐ Whole words only <br> ☐ First Author only | <br> ☐ Ignore case <br> ☐ Whole words only |
| | Min. frequency | 6 | 1 |
| | Diagrams | ☑ Top 8  scaled with auto ▾ | |
| | Details | ☑ alphabetically ▾ ascending ▾  ☐ Show always PMID | |
| | MeSH codes | ☐ | |
| Output | MeSH tree | ☑ Print depth 10 <br> F: Psychiatry and Psychology ▾ <br> as preferred branch to collect frequencies | |
| | Link restrictor | Optical Illusions[mh] 2000 [dp] | |
| | Data format | HTML ▾ | |
| | Comment | My first search | |
| | File name | Optical_illusions[mh]_2000[dp].txt  Choose | |

Consult Meva  Clear

Fig. 2. Meva's consultation form

Meva provides a context-sensitive help for all form parameters by clicking on their names. Besides, help files assist in the usage of Meva and its analysis results.

**Filters and Minimal Frequencies.** Users can specify search filters or minimal frequencies to restrict Meva's analysis radius. In this example, the user limited Meva's processing to terms with a minimal frequency of six and to MeSH major topics (containing an asterisk). Boolean operators can be used in filter expressions as well like OR, AND or NOT. Searching for authors can be limited to first authors.

**Diagrams.** With these parameters, field count and scaling of Meva's histograms and correlation matrices can be adjusted (here: eight most frequent fields chosen).

**Details.** These parameters control the sorting type and order for the details table.

**MeSH Codes.** The user may decide to display the codes of the MeSH terms.

**MeSH Tree.** All MeSH terms of the PubMed result as can be displayed as a hierarchical tree. The tree depth (here: 10) and other parameters can be adjusted as well.

**Link Restrictor.** Passing the original search expression used in PubMed into this input box allows Meva to link its analysis result with PubMed. Clicking onto one of the field values in Meva's analysis result will trigger a new search in PubMed for the value of the clicked field plus the value of the link restrictor box. Thus a stepwise refinement of the original search can be easily performed in an interactive way.

**Result Format.** The resulting output can be delivered as HTML or in a delimited format to import into a database of the users choice.

### 2.3  Meva's Preprocessing

PubMed's result file can be compressed before sending it to Meva by MePrep, the Meva preprocessor. Thus the net traffic load can be decreased and the processing speed of client and server can be increased. This procedure is recommended for input file sizes larger than five MB. Compression rates between 5 to 80% can be achieved.

### 2.4  Meva's Output

Meva displays its analysis result showing a graphical condensed representation of counts and relations of the bibliographic fields. It uses histograms, correlation tables, a detailed sorted list and a MeSH tree. MeSH codes for MeSH terms may be listed. If the user provided a link restrictor in Meva's consultation form, the displayed field values are linked: a click onto a field triggers a new search in PubMed. The following sections illustrate details of the Meva result from the example input mentioned above.

**Totals.** The header of each Meva result includes a totals table indicating the count of the bibliographic fields at all processing stages of the analysis (Fig. 3).

**Total**

| Phase | Article | MeSH Term | Author |
|---|---|---|---|
| Read in | 108 | 1010 | 269 |
| Passed the filters | | 344 | 269 |
| Identified as distinct | | 116 | 247 |
| Minimal frequencies reached and admitted to database | | 11 | 247 |

**Fig. 3.** Meva's totals table output

**Histograms.** Meva displays a histogram of the most frequent values (top values) per each selected bibliographic field. Fig. 4 shows the 1st histogram of two.

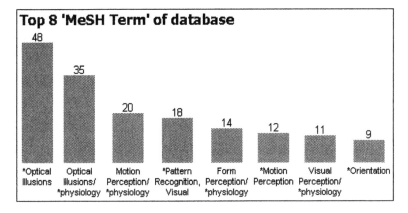

**Fig. 4.** Meva's histogram output for the eight *top MeSH terms*

**Correlation Matrices.** These tables show the coincidence between the top values of the 1st field and between those of the 1st and the 2nd field. Fig. 5 shows the 2nd table.

## Coincidence Top 'MeSH Term' - Top 'Author'

|  | Cavanagh P | Whitney D | Shimojo S | Murakami I | Krekelberg B | Proffitt DR | Popple AV | Pavlova M | Total |
|---|---|---|---|---|---|---|---|---|---|
| *Optical Illusions | 1 | 1 | 1 |  | 1 | 1 |  | 1 | 6 |
| Optical Illusions/ *physiology | 3 | 1 | 1 | 1 | 1 |  | 2 |  | 9 |
| Motion Perception/ *physiology | 4 | 2 | 1 | 2 | 1 |  |  | 1 | 11 |
| *Pattern Recognition, Visual |  |  |  |  |  | 2 |  |  | 2 |
| Form Perception/ *physiology |  |  |  |  |  |  |  |  | 0 |
| *Motion Perception | 1 | 1 | 1 |  | 1 |  |  | 1 | 5 |
| Visual Perception/ *physiology |  |  | 1 |  |  |  | 1 |  | 2 |
| *Orientation |  |  |  |  |  | 2 |  |  | 2 |
| Total | 9 | 5 | 5 | 3 | 4 | 5 | 3 | 3 | 37 |

**Fig. 5.** Meva's correlation matrix output for the eight *top MeSH terms* and *top authors*

**Details Table.** Apart from the diagrams, Meva's details table shows the values of all selected bibliographic fields with the PMID for article retrieval in PubMed (Fig. 6).

## Details of database

| i | nc | n | MeSH Term | PMID | Author |
|---|----|----|-----------|------|--------|
| 1 | 7 | 7 | *Attention | 11273404 | Suzuki S, Peterson MA |
| | | | | 11273385 | Crawford LE, Huttenlocher J, Engebretson PH |
| | | | | 11153859 | Kincade S, Wilson AE |
| | | | | 11143444 | Palmer SE, Nelson R |
| | | | | 11131742 | Gunn DV, Warm JS, Dember WN, Temple JG |
| | | | | 11114232 | Servos P, Carnahan H, Fedwick J |
| | | | | 10997045 | Sokolov A, Pavlova M, Ehrenstein WH |
| 2 | 19 | 12 | *Motion Perception | 11273404 | Suzuki S, Peterson MA |
| | | | | 11219985 | Sheth BR, Shimojo S |
| | | | | 11184992 | Patel SS, Ogmen H, Bedell HE, Sampath V |

**Fig. 6.** Meva's details table output (detail only)

**MeSH Tree.** If the user selected MeSH terms in Meva's form, a tree of all MeSH terms along with their codes and cumulated frequencies will be displayed (Fig. 7).

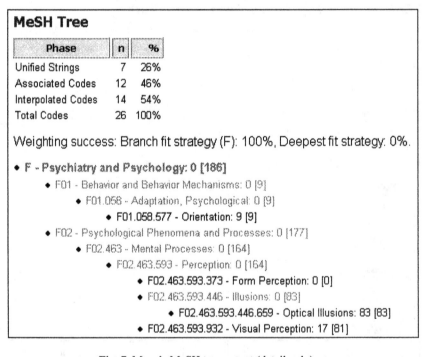

## MeSH Tree

| Phase | n | % |
|-------|----|------|
| Unified Strings | 7 | 26% |
| Associated Codes | 12 | 46% |
| Interpolated Codes | 14 | 54% |
| Total Codes | 26 | 100% |

Weighting success: Branch fit strategy (F): 100%, Deepest fit strategy: 0%.

- F - Psychiatry and Psychology: 0 [186]
    - F01 - Behavior and Behavior Mechanisms: 0 [9]
        - F01.058 - Adaptation, Psychological: 0 [9]
            - F01.058.577 - Orientation: 9 [9]
    - F02 - Psychological Phenomena and Processes: 0 [177]
        - F02.463 - Mental Processes: 0 [164]
            - F02.463.593 - Perception: 0 [164]
                - F02.463.593.373 - Form Perception: 0 [0]
                - F02.463.593.446 - Illusions: 0 [83]
                    - F02.463.593.446.659 - Optical Illusions: 83 [83]
                - F02.463.593.932 - Visual Perception: 17 [81]

**Fig. 7.** Meva's MeSH tree output (detail only)

# 3  Benefit of Meva

Meva's facilitates the evaluation of PubMed's results by displaying a well-structured expressive result. Histograms, correlation tables, detailed sorted lists and MeSH trees allow a condensed representation of PubMed's data.

## 3.1  General Advantages

Meva is available *world-wide* by its web interface (currently at http://www.med-ai.com/meva/). Its usage is now *free of charge* since the service is based upon PubMed. Meva can be installed on any HTTP1.1/CGI1.1/multipart-form-data compliant web server [2; 6]. Acting as a server-based program, Meva can be maintained in a *centralized way*. There is no need for an installation of a client-based retrieval software: only a HTML4/CSS1 compliant *standard web browser* is required. Analysis can be heavily *customized* by the user through the consultation form by selecting, filtering and cross-relating bibliographic fields of interest. By supplying PubMed links inside Meva's result, users are able to *refine* their original search stepwise in a convenient way. Results can be printed out, used off-line for *presentations* [5] and *statistical evaluations* or imported into a *database*.

## 3.2  Specific Advantages

Histograms assist in finding the *most important values* of a selected bibliographic field. Thus question like "Which author has the most publications in a special area?" or "Which therapeutic approach is used most often?" can be answered by Meva. Besides, histograms can be used to obtain a *quick synopsis* of a medical topic.

Correlation matrices facilitate the findings of important *relations* between bibliographic fields, e.g. country - affiliation, country - author, affiliation - MeSH term, author - MeSH term etc. Questions like "Which therapeutical approach gives the best results?" can be answered easier this way. Medical laymen can gain helpful information as well. A typical question could be "Where does the specialist for a certain disease live and what is his name?" (correlation author - MeSH term, author - affiliation). *Author profiles* can be derived using this classification procedure. *First authors* can be extracted. The combination of a bibliographic field with the publication date field allows an illustration of the progress of this field *in time*, e.g. the evolution of MeSH terms or the main publishing period of authors.

In contradiction to PubMed's MeSH browser, Meva builds a MeSH tree for all MeSH terms of the PubMed result. This allows the user to identify *additional significant key words* for a refined PubMed search. With the help of PubMed's clinical filters along with Meva's MeSH features, the user can efficiently obtain valuable patient-oriented evidence that matters, POEM called with regard to the EBM movement [4]. Due to the fact that MeSH multiplies the usefulness of the MEDLINE database and makes it possible to search the medical literature as we do today [1], the MeSH tree feature can assist in a professional search.

## 3.3  Conclusion

The development of Meva marks a clear progress in the fields of data mining in MEDLINE. This service extends the capabilities of the PubMed user interface by far and represents a huge advancement in the retrieval of hidden knowledge in the world's largest medical library.

# References

1. Coletti, M.H., Bleich, H.L.: Medical Subject Headings Used to Search the Biomedical Literature. J. Am. Med. Inform. Assoc. 8 (2001) 317–323
2. Kientzle, T.: Internet-Dateiformate - Windows, DOS, UNIX & Mac. 1st edn International Thomson Publishing, Bonn (1996)
3. Lusti, M.: Data Warehousing und Data Mining: Eine Einführung in entscheidungsunterstützende Systeme. 2nd edn Springer-Verlag, Berlin Heidelberg New York (2002)
4. Shaughnessy, A.F., Slawson, D.C., Bennett, J.H.: Becoming an information master: a guidebook to the medical information jungle. J. Fam. Pract. 39 (1994) 489-499
5. Thurmayr, G.R., Thurmayr, R., Tenner, H., Ingenerf, J.: Womit beschäftigt sich zur Zeit die Med. Informatik? Eine MEDLINE-Analyse. Informatik, Biometrie und Epidemiologie in Medizin und Biologie 33 (2002) 100
6. Tischer, M., Jennrich, B.: Internet intern - Technik und Programmierung. 1st edn Data-Becker-Verlag, Düsseldorf (1997)

# Isobologram Analysis in MATLAB for Combined Effects of Two Agents in Dose-Response Experiments

Stefan Wagenpfeil[1], Uwe Treiber[2], and Antonie Lehmer[2]

[1] Institut für Medizinische Statistik und Epidemiologie der Technischen Universität München, Klinikum rechts der Isar, Ismaninger Str. 22,
D-81675 München, Germany
stefan.wagenpfeil@imse.med.tu-muenchen.de
http://www.imse.med.tu-muenchen.de/persons/wagenpfeil/index.html
[2] Urologische Klinik und Poliklinik der Technischen Universität München,
Klinikum rechts der Isar, Ismaninger Str. 22,
D-81675 München, Germany

**Abstract.** Isobologram analysis is a way of exploring and visualizing combined drug effects. The aim of this work is to determine as to whether two agents can be considered synergistic or antagonistic. Resulting from a clinical consulting case in urology we developed a MATLAB-based software tool for automated isobologram analysis. In this way we supplement the clinical software-equipment in our laboratory and encourage the evaluation of combined dose-response experiments. Analysis of an example data set demonstrates the approach and the way of interpreting obtained results.

## 1 Introduction

In the laboratory department of the Urologische Klinik und Poliklinik der Technischen Universität München, Klinikum rechts der Isar, the potential inhibition of prostate tumor cell lines with specific retinoids and taxans is examined in vitro. After dealing with one-agent experiments and exploring dose-response effects with increasing concentrations and decreasing cell survival rates [1], the combined effect of two drugs on the outcome cell survival rate is now of interest. Concentrations are usually measured in $\mu$M or nM, starting with small values and increasing accordingly. Response rates are obtained by ELISA (enzymelinked immunosorbent assay)-reading ranging from 100% to 0% cell survival rate. In general, 42 and up to 225 or more dose combinations of two agents are examined in one trial and therefore a respective number of dose-response values are obtained. Table 1 displays an example file from Dr. Kano (see acknowledgement) for the combined effect of a particular agent A (concentration measured in $\mu$M) and agent B (concentration measured in nM) on a prespecified tumor cell line. Agent A may be a retinoid and B a taxan.

P. Perner et al. (Eds.): ISMDA 2003, LNCS 2868, pp. 47–54, 2003.

**Table 1.** Example data on cell survival rates in % depending on different combinations of drug concentrations A[$\mu$M] and B[nM].

| A \ B | 0 [nM] | 5 [nM] | 10 [nM] | 15 [nM] | 20 [nM] | 30[nM] |
|---|---|---|---|---|---|---|
| 0 [$\mu$M] | 100 | 88 | 65 | 50 | 32 | 17 |
| 0.1 [$\mu$M] | 92 | 77 | 58 | 45 | 26 | 16 |
| 0.2 [$\mu$M] | 84 | 65 | 49 | 37 | 23 | 15 |
| 0.5 [$\mu$M] | 61 | 47 | 38 | 30 | 18 | 10 |
| 1 [$\mu$M] | 39 | 33 | 25 | 19 | 14 | 7 |
| 2 [$\mu$M] | 26 | 23 | 18 | 14 | 9 | 6 |
| 5 [$\mu$M] | 10 | 9 | 8 | 5 | 5 | 3 |

Looking at the rows we can see that survival rates decrease with increasing concentrations of drug B. The baseline value and the strength of decrease depends on the additional concentration of drug A.

A basis for statistical inference on combined drug effects is the estimation of the underlying "true" dose-response relationship for either drug, which is a classical problem discussed in more detail e.g. in [2]. A common approach for exploring connections of the present kind with continuous doses and scaled binomial outcomes is the 4-parameter logistic regression model as a generalized version of the log-logit model. Due to uncertainties in laboratory measurements, upper and lower bounds of response rates cannot be fixed in advance when evaluating real data sets. In order to take uncertainties about lower and upper bounds of response rates into account we prefer the 4-parameter logistic rather than the log-logit model. The model equation is specified by

$$y = \frac{a - d}{1 + (\frac{x}{c})^b} + d \, , \tag{1}$$

where $y$ is the estimated cell survival rate at concentration $x$. As we have, from a theoretical point of view, a 100% cell survival for concentration $x = 0$ and a low survival rate for sufficiently high values of $x$ in our case, a natural choice for $a$ and $d$ in (1) is $a = 1$ and $d = 0$. This yields the log-logit model. Parameter $b$ describes how rapidly the survival curve makes its transition from the asymptotes to the center of the curve, and $c$ is the 50% concentration (concentration with 50% survival rate) to be estimated.

The 4-parameter logistic regression model fits into the well-known class of nonlinear regression models. 95% confidence intervals (CI) can be obtained along the lines given in [1]. Fig. 1 and Fig. 2 display the resulting dose-response curves for either drug from Table 1 on a semilog scale.

Concentrations $10^{-5}$ nM and $10^{-5}$ $\mu$M instead of 0 nM and 0 $\mu$M were choosen in the analysis for numerical reasons, respectively.

The effect of a two-agent combination on cell survival rates in vitro from the example data is analyzed in the following by two-dimensional isobolograms originally described by Steel and Peckham [3] and manually used by Kano et al.

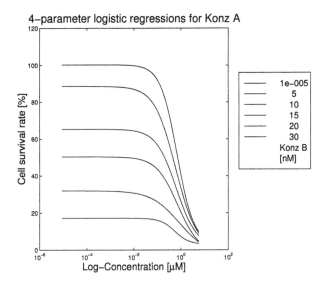

**Fig. 1.** Dose-response curves (—) for drug A

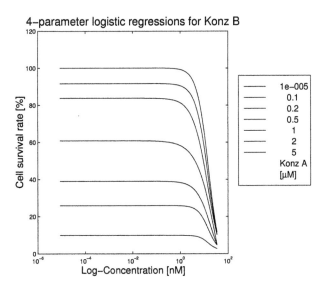

**Fig. 2.** Dose-response curves (—) for drug B

for anti-cancer agents in culture [4]. In the next section we describe a method for automated and computerized isobologram analysis and address computational issues. Following the results section we conclude with general remarks on interpreting graphical displays of isobolograms, essential issues for implementing isobologram routines and a reference to high-dimensional isobolograms.

## 2  Methods for Data Analysis

An isobologram is a graphical output consisting of two parts: A two-dimensional scatterplot of combinations of inhibitory concentrations and an envelope of additivity determined by mode I and mode II additivity lines. Fig. 3 displays an example of an inhibitory concentration (IC) 50 isobologram.

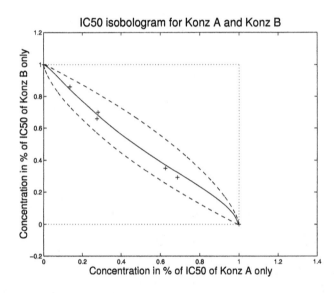

**Fig. 3.** IC50 isobologram for agents A and B. (+) are IC50 combinations, (—) is the mode I additivity line and (- -) the envelope of additivity from mode II

ICp is defined as the p% inhibitory concentration for a specific agent, that is p% of tumor celles are inhibited by the agent at concentration ICp yielding a cell survival rate of (1-p)%. If p=80, the IC80 concentration belongs to a cell survival rate of 20%. In the following we focus on IC80 concentrations.

IC80 concentrations are conveniently obtained in two steps: First estimate the parameters $a$, $b$, $c$ and $d$ of a 4-parameter logistic regression model (1) along with respective 95% CI's. Secondly insert the resulting parameter estimates in the inverse formula of (1) given by

$$x = c\left(\frac{a - y}{y - d}\right)^{1/b} .$$ 

(2)

Setting y=100-80=20 yields x=IC80. In our example the IC80 values of agents A and B can be captured from Fig. 1 and 2. For isobologram display, concentration values are scaled relative to IC80 thus ranging from 0 to 1.

The isobologram envelope lines can solely be computed from dose-response curves of agent A (Fig. 4) and B (Fig. 5) out of uncombined experiments.

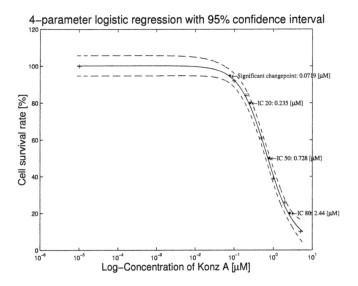

**Fig. 4.** Dose-response curve for agent A with logscaled abscissa. (+) observed data, (—) estimated response curve, (- -) pointwise 95% CI

Significant changepoints indicate a significant reduction in cell survival rates [1], but are of no further concern here.

A mode I additivity line shows combinations of drug concentrations in circumstances of hetero-additive combined drug effects. They can be calculated as follows: Define a grid from 0 to IC80 for agent A, for instance. Compute for each of the grid points the fraction inhibited F out of Fig. 4. Determine the concentration of agent B needed out of Fig. 5 in order to obtain a cell survival rate of 20%+F using equation (2).

Iso-additive combined drug effects are shown by mode II additivity lines. The procedure is as follows: Define a grid from 0 to IC80 for agent A, for instance. Compute for each of the grid points the fraction inhibited F out of Fig. 4. Determine the concentration of agent B needed to come down to a cell survival rate of 20% starting with IC(1-F) on the dose-response curve of drug B, cf. Fig. 5. This is obtained by calculating IC80-IC(1-F) with IC values from drug B and conveniently using equation (2) again. Let (s,t) be the coordinates of the resulting additivity line in the plane. Then (1-s, 1-t) are the coordinates of the corresponding second iso-additive line.

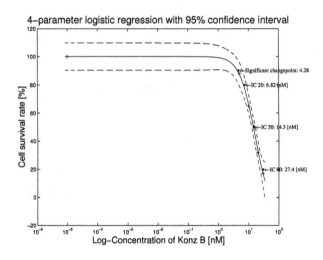

**Fig. 5.** Dose-response curve for agent B with logscaled abscissa. (+) observed data, (—) estimated response curve, (- -) pointwise 95% CI

As we do not know whether the combined drug effect we examine will be iso-additive, hetero-additive or intermediate, all possibilities should be considered. All of these features are implemented in a MATLAB-based software tool IBG. The following section shows the results obtained with IBG.

## 3    Results

Estimated inhibitory concentrations IC50, IC80 and % of IC80 from 4-parameter logistic regression (1) and inverse formula (2) along with respective 95% CI's are given in Table 2 and 3 for agent A and B, respectively. An IC-value of zero means an inhibition of 80% is already obtained and therefore the respective agent is not necessary any more in this setting. The short cut inf for infinity on the right side of a confidence interval indicates an interval that is unbounded from above.

Fig. 6 displays the resulting IC80 isobologram for our example data given in Table 1. We can see that all IC combinations of agent A and B lie inside the envelope of additivity. Thus in combination they have an additive effect on the outcome cell survival.

## 4    Conclusion

From an isobologram we can see immediately the effect of a combination of two drugs and the way they act: synergistic, additive or antagonistic. An effect is called additive if the data points in the isobologram representing estimated IC combinations fall mainly within the envelope of additivity. When the data points fall below the area of additivity, the combination is considered supra-additive or

**Table 2.** Estimated IC's with [95% CI] for agent A and different concentrations of agent B.

| B[nM] | IC50 | IC80 | % of IC80 |
|---|---|---|---|
| 0 | 0.73 [0.64 ... 0.83] | 2.44 [1.98 ... 3.2] | 1 [0.81 ... 1.31] |
| 5 | 0.46 [0.38 ... 0.54] | 2.12 [1.67 ... 2.81] | 0.87 [0.69 ... 1.15] |
| 10 | 0.2 [0.15 ... 0.26] | 1.54 [1.21 ... 1.96] | 0.63 [0.5 ... 0.8] |
| 15 | 0 [0 ... 0.06] | 1.03 [0.76 ... 1.44] | 0.42 [0.31 ... 0.59] |
| 20 | 0 [0 ... 0] | 0.36 [0.32 ... 0.39] | 0.15 [0.13 ... 0.16] |
| 30 | 0 [0 ... 0] | 0 [0 ... 0] | 0 [0 ... 0] |

**Table 3.** Estimated IC's with [95% CI] for agent B and different concentrations of agent A.

| A[$\mu$M] | IC50 | IC80 | % of IC80 |
|---|---|---|---|
| 0 | 14.29 [12.44 ... 16.52] | 27.43 [23.46 ... inf] | 1 [0.86 ... inf] |
| 0.1 | 12.31 [9.3 ... 15.92] | 25.8 [19.76 ... inf] | 0.94 [0.72 ... inf] |
| 0.2 | 9.42 [6.9 ... 11.99] | 24.25 [19.18 ... inf] | 0.88 [0.7 ... inf] |
| 0.5 | 4.17 [0.04 ... 7.49] | 20.55 [15.45 ... inf] | 0.75 [0.56 ... inf] |
| 1 | 0 [0 ... 0] | 14.05 [13.51 ... 14.66] | 0.51 [0.49 ... 0.53] |
| 2 | 0 [0 ... 0] | 8.15 [5.36 ... 10.41] | 0.3 [0.2 ... 0.38] |
| 5 | 0 [0 ... 0] | 0 [0 ... 0] | 0 [0 ... 0] |

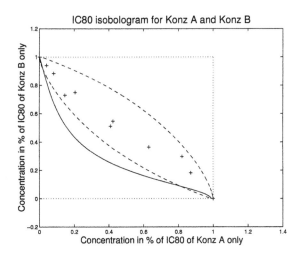

**Fig. 6.** IC80 isobologram for agents A and B

synergistic. When the data points fall above the envelope, the combined effect is regarded as antagonistic. For more details see [5]. From 95% CI's as given in Tables 2 and 3 for IC-values statistical significance as well as accuracy or uncertainty of estimates can be derived. In particular they can be used to determine the significance of synergism or antagonism, cf. [5,6].

For the implementation a lot of error code has to be written since there are many possibilities for unregularities in the data or estimates of infinity. From a numerical point of view there should be enough data as we are in a 2-dimensional space (input data in matrix form as in Table 1). Moreover nonlinear regression (1) needs a sufficiently high number of observations. More extensive datasets are in preparation in our laboratory and valuable tools for applying the regression model (1) are contained in the optimization toolbox of MATLAB [7].

In order to evaluate the effect of more than two agents we can think of 3- or higher-dimensional isobolograms. However, only 3-dimensional isobolograms can be displayed as given in [5]. Although we may analyse effects of more than three agents there is no way of drawing isobolograms with more than three dimensions.

*Acknowledgement:* Personal communication with Dr. Kano, Tochigi Cancer Center, Utsunomiya, Japan, is gratefully acknowledged. We thank Dr. Kano for providing these illuminating example data.

# References

1. Wagenpfeil, S., Treiber, U., Lehmer, A.: A MATLAB-Based Software Tool for Changepoint Detection and Nonlinear Regression in Dose-Response Relationships, *in* Medical Data Analysis (Brause, R.W., Hanisch, E., eds.), Lecture Notes in Computer Science Vol. 1993, Springer-Verlag, Berlin (2000) 190–197
2. Chuang-Stein, C., Agresti, A.: Tutorial in Biostatistics: A Review of Tests for Detecting a Monotone Dose-Response Relationship with Ordinal Response Data. Statistics in Medicine **16** (1997) 2599–2618
3. Steel, G.G., Peckham, M.J.: Exploitable mechanisms in combined radiotherapy-chemotherapy: the concept of additivity. Int. J. Radiat. Oncol. Biol. Physiol. **5** (1979) 85–91
4. Kano, Y., Suzuki, K., Akutsu, M., Suda, K., Inoue, Y., Yoshida, M., Sakamoto, S., Miura, Y.: Effects of CPT-11 in combination with other anti-cancer agents in culture. Int. J. Cancer **50** (1992) 604–610
5. Nashizaki, M., Meyn, R.E., Levy, L.B., Atkinson, E.N., White, R.A., Roth, J.A., Ji, L.: Synergistic Inhibition of Human Lung Cancer Cell Growth by Adenovirus-mediated Wild-Type p53 Gene Transfer in Combination with Docetaxel and Radiation Therapeutics in Vitro and in Vivo. Clin Cancer Res **7** (2001) 2887–2897
6. Kano, Y., Akutsu, M., Suzuki, K., Mori, K., Yazawa, Y., Tsunoda, S.: Schedule-dependent interactions between paclitaxel and etoposide in human carcinoma cell lines in vitro. Cancer Chemother Pharmacol **44** (1999) 381–388
7. Coleman, Th., Branch, M.A., Grace, A.: Optimization Toolbox for Use with MAT-LAB, User's Guide, Version 2. 3rd printing, The Math Works Inc., Natick, MA 01760-1500, USA (1999)

# Towards an Improved On-line Algorithm to Estimate the Fetal Heart Rate from Ultrasound Data

Martin Daumer[1], Christian Harböck[1], Felix Ko[1], Christian Lederer[1], Thomas Schindler[1,2], and Michael Scholz[1]

[1] Trium Analysis Online GmbH
c/o Institute for Medical Statistics and Epidemiology
Klinikum r.d. Isar Ismaninger Str. 22 81675 München Germany
[2] Institute for Medical Statistics and Epidemiology
Klinikum r.d. Isar Ismaninger Str. 22 81675 München Germany

**Abstract.** We describe a new algorithm which estimates the fetal heart rate from ultrasound data. First comparisons show its potential to give a more reliable estimate of the true fetal heart rate than the algorithms embedded in standard CTG (cardio-toco-graphy) monitoring devices.

## Introduction

For a long time, the fetal movements observed by the mother were the only possibility to obtain information about the health of the unborn child. At the beginning of the 19th century the importance of measuring the fetal heart beat via stethoscope was perceived, and this method continued to be the only established monitoring tool until about 40 years ago. The cornerstone for the present standard method of cardiotocography (CTG) using the Doppler effect in ultrasound measurements of the fetal heart was laid by Hammacher [1] at the beginning of the sixties with essential contributions of Saling [2] and Hon [3]. During just a few years, the CTG was introduced as a standard into medical practice. By means of a CTG visualization the obstetrician or the midwife tries to judge, weather the fetal health is compromised. There exists a variety of rules and scoring systems, e.g. [4], [5] and FIGO (international federation for gynecology and obstetrics) [6], which should allow to classify CTG traces in a meaningful and prognostically relevant way.

Nevertheless, it is well-known that the CTG is related with a high inter- and intraobserver variability and has a high rate of false positive alarms, i.e. when the CTG is considered to be pathological although the fetus is in good health. Some authors argue that this has led to an increased rate of unnecessary cesarian sections, see [7], [8], [9].

There are various ways how to improve that situation: using an algorithm to detect patterns in the fetal heart rate, using an algorithm to generate an graded

P. Perner et al. (Eds.): ISMDA 2003, LNCS 2868, pp. 55–61, 2003.

alarm depending on the various patterns and using an intenet-based user-interface which allows to bring the right information to the decision-maker faster. We have developed a system which reads preprocessed fetal heart rate (FHR) data from standard CTG monitoring devices. It contains an automatic on-line pattern recognition in the fetal heart rate (based on the delayed moving windows algorithm [10]), an on-line expert system based on the rules of the FIGO [6] and an internet-based graphical user interface. "Trium CTG Online" is now a CE-certified medical product and is successfully running in some German hospitals.

However, the system relies upon the correctness of the estimates of the true FHR given by the CTG monitoring devices. Although the basic principle using the autocorrelation function seems to be the basis in all CTG monitoring devices on the market, considerable differences between the CTG monitoring devices can be observed. Moreover, an overall tendency of "smoothing" the fetal heart rate seems to have become more pronounced over the years and may lead to the display of heart rate patterns with a low variablity which is usually considered to be pathological, thus leading to an increase in the rate of false alarms [9].

In this paper we describe a new algorithm which estimates the fetal heart rate from ultrasound data. First comparisons show its potential to give a more reliable estimate of the true fetal heart rate than the algorithms embedded in standard CTG monitoring devices.

## 1   Methods

Figure 1 shows a typical "well-behaved" raw US signal (approx. 1.4 seconds). "Well-behaved" means, that the fetal heart beat (FHR) is clearly audible using a loudspeaker and also clearly visible which is both the case in Fig. 1.

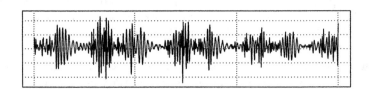

**Fig. 1.** "Well-behaved" raw ultrasound (US) signal

The usual strategy for calculating the fetal heart beat rate is as follows:

1. Calculate a "hull curve" from the modulus of the US signal.

2. Calculate the autocorrelation function (ACF) for this hull curve.

3. Calculate the heart beat rate from the maximum of the ACF.

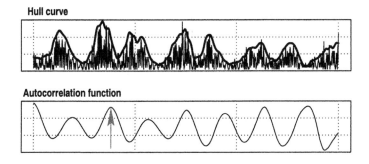

**Fig. 2.** Hull curve of a US signal and corresponding ACF. Even an US signal of very high quality may generate an ACF with many local maxima. The maximum corresponding to the fetal heart rate is marked by the arrow.

The disadvantages of this approach are obvious: The hull curve hides a lot of information from the raw signal, namely the frequency change during a typical heart action, which is clearly audibly for the human ear. Thus, the hull curve cannot distinguish very well between different parts of a single heart action. This leads to an autocorrelation function with many local maxima, where it is difficult to decide which corresponds to the fetal heart beat rate (the right one is marked with the green arrow in the above figure).

One should also notice, that US signal may contain pieces of noise, which appear as "scratches" to the human ear (see Fig. 3). These scratches usually totally disturb the above algorithm.

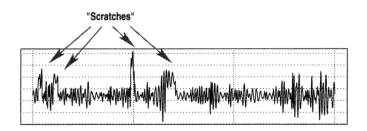

**Fig. 3.** Noisy US signal

The basic idea of our algorithm is to consider the US signal as an essentially frequency modulated signal. Thus we use a moving FFT window in order to detect raises of frequencies which are characteristic for specific parts of one single heart action.

- The autocorrelation functions for the single frequencies typically have much less local maxima, since they cannot confuse different parts of two heart actions.

- Often noise affects only a part of the heart action. Hence, removing noisy parts of the US signal (i.e. considering them as missing values), will in most cases at most affect a single frequency.

- The improved robustness against noise enable us to calculate the FHR from smaller time windows. This again makes the algorithm more sensitive to sudden FHR changes, which are a major problem for all currently used FHR algorithms (see [9]).

- The "agreement" between several autocorrelation functions can be used in order to estimate the quality of the US signal and the reliability of the calculated FHR.

Another idea of our algorithm is the intentional use of noise: In order to calculate the ACF for incomplete time series, a straight forward application of the fast Fourier transformation (FFT) is not possible. However, using a "dumb" method for calculating the ACF would be computationally not feasible. The idea was to impute appropriate noise for the missings. The right way to do this was to impute a bootstrap sample from the available data for the missings. This automatically has the right range and does not introduce artefact into the ACF, since the imputed values do not correlate. Figure 4 shows a schematic flow diagram of the algorithm.

## 2   Results

As a first step towards validation of the new algorithm the fetal heart rate estimates were compared with the estimates from a standard CTG monitoring device (see Fig. 6). For that we used parallel recordings of the ultrasound raw data and the output of a standard CTG device. The raw data were then transformed into fetal heart rate estimates offline using the new algorithm and were compared visually with the standard.

A closer inspection of raw data and corresponding estimated fetal heart rate suggests, that the algorithm above seems be be more robust against noisy data, and seems to be more sensitive against sudden changes in the FHR.

## 3   Discussion

The findings suggest that the new algorithm leads to the same estimates of the fetal heart rate as a standard monitoring device when there is a good signal quality and no rapid changes in the fetal heart rate. For noisy signals and rapid

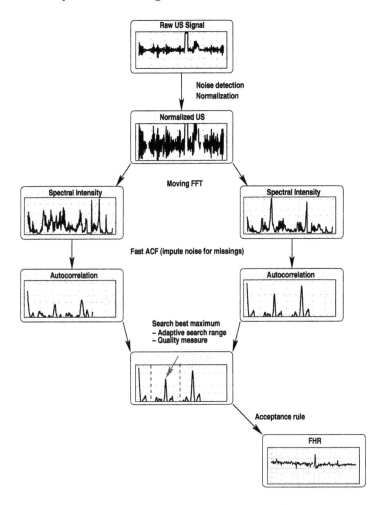

**Fig. 4.** Flow diagram of the algorithm

changes in the fetal heart rate the new algorithm may have the potential to give more reliable estimates. Further fine-tuning of parameters using a variety of different US recordings will probably lead to improvements but eventually one has to compare the new algorithm and the standard methods with some sort of "gold standard". The natural choice is given by the extraction of the fetal heart rate from (invasive) recordings of the fetal electrocardiogram in order to see whether there is a "real" improvement in the estimate. Such an improvement could be of high relevance for the entire field of CTG monitoring [9].

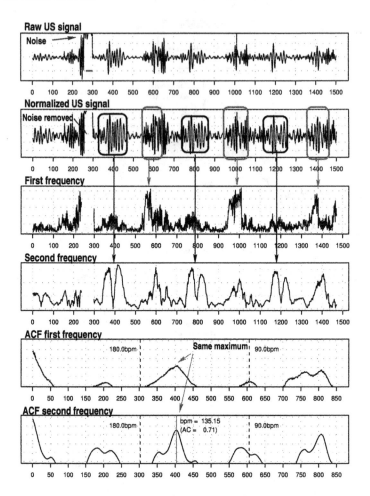

**Fig. 5.** Analysis of a typical US sequence

# References

[1] Hammacher, K., Werners, P.: On the evaluation and documentation of ctg (cardiotocographic) results. Gynaecologia **165** (1968) 410–423

[2] Saling, E., Dudenhausen, J.: The present situation of clinical monitoring of the fetus during labor. J. Perinat. Med. **1** (1973) 75–103

[3] Hon, E.: The electronic evaluation of the fetal heart rate. Am. J. Obstet. Gynecol. **75** (1958) 1215–1230

[4] Fischer, W., Stude, I., Brandt, H.: A suggestion for the evaluation of the antepartal cardiotocogram. Z. Geburtshilfe. Perinatol. **180** (1976) 117–123

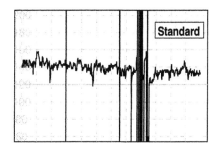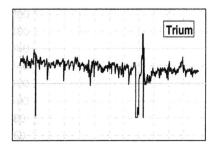

**Fig. 6.** FHR plots for qualitative comparison between a standard CTG device and the new algorithm using a typical section of a long recording. Vertical lines indicate values our of range.

[5] Krebs et al., H.: Intrapartum fetal heart rate monitoring. Am. J. Obstet. Gynecol. **133** (1979) 762–772

[6] Rooth, G., Huch, A., Huch, R.: Figo news: Guidelines for the use of fetal monitoring. Int. J. Gynaecol. Obstet. **25** (1987) 159–167

[7] Impey et al., L.: Admission cardiotocography: a randomised controlled trial. Lancet (2003) 465–470

[8] Thacker, S., Stroup, D.: Revisiting the use of the electronic fetal monitor. Lancet (2003) 445–446

[9] Morgenstern, J., Abels, T., Hollbrügge, P., Somville, T., Weis, G., P.Wolf: CTG-Geräte Test '93. Technical report, Medizinische Einrichtungen der Heinrich-Heine-Universität Düsseldorf (1994)

[10] Daumer, M.: Method and device for detecting drifts, jumps and/or outliers of measurement values. US Patent No. US 8,556,957 B1 (2003)

[11] Lighthill, M.: Introduction to Fourier Analysis and Generalized Functions. Cambridge University Press (1962)

[12] Efron, B., Tibshirani, R.: An Introduction to the Bootstrap. Number 57 in Monographs on Statistics and Applied Probability. Chapman & Hall/CRC (1998)

# Health Monitoring by an Image Interpretation System – A System for Airborne Fungi Identification

P. Perner[1], T. Günther[2], H. Perner[1], G. Fiss[1], R. Ernst[1]

[1] Institute of Computer Vision and Applied Computer Sciences
Körnerstr. 10, 04107 Leipzig
ibaiperner@aol.com
http:// www.ibai-research.de
[2] JenaBios GmbH, Loebstedter Str. 78
D-07749 Jena

**Abstract.** Human beings are exposed every day to bioaerosols in the various fields of their personal and/or professional daily life. The European Commission has rules protecting employees in the workplace from biological hazards. Airborne fungi can be detected and identified by an image acquisition and interpretation system. In this paper we present recent results on the development of an image interpretation system for airborne fungi identification. We explain the application domain and describe the development issues. The development strategy and the architecture of the system are described. Finally we give recent results and an outlook to future work.

## 1 Introduction

Airborne microorganisms are ubiquitous present the various fields of indoor and outdoor environments. The potential implication of fungal contaminants in bioaerosols on occupational health is recognized as a problem in several working environments. There is concern on exposure of workers to bioaerosols especially in composting facilities, in agriculture and in municipal waste treatment. At the moment it is assumed that in the Federal Republic of Germany in 20% of the workplaces it has been discovered a negative influence by biological agents. Potentially endangered could be 8 million employees. The European Commission has therefore guiding rules protecting employees in the workplace from airborne biological hazards.

Despite this there is an increasing number of incidents for building-related sickness, especially in office and residential building. Some of these problems are attributed to biological agents especial to airborne fungal spores. However, the knowledge of health effects of indoor fungal contaminants is still restricted since appropriate methods for rapid and long-time monitoring of airborne microorganisms are not available.

Besides the detection of parameters relevant to occupational and public health, in many controlled environments the number of airborne microorganisms has to be kept below the permissible or recommended values (e.g. clean rooms, operating theaters, domains of the food and pharmaceutical industry) [1].

P. Perner et al. (Eds.): ISMDA 2003, LNCS 2868, pp. 62-74, 2003.
© Springer-Verlag Berlin Heidelberg 2003

The continuous monitoring of airborne biological agents is consequently a necessity, as well for the detection of risks for human health as for the smooth sequence of technological processes.

At present a variety of methods for detection of fungal spores is frequently used. The culture-based methods depend on growth of spores on an agar plate and counting of colony forming units. Culture-independent methods are based on the enumeration of spores under a microscope or uses the polymerase chain reaction or DNA hybridization for detection of fungi. However, all methods are limited by time-consuming procedures of sample preparation in the laboratory.

Aim of the project is the development and realisation of an image-acquisition unit of biologically dangerous substances and the automatic analysis of these images. The basic principle of the system shall lie in that dust and bio-aerosols are conducted in defined volumina via special carrying agents and separated there, that they are registered by an image-acquisition unit, counted, classified and that their nature is defined, by means of an automatic image-interpretation system.

The variability of the biological objects is very broad and the constraints of the image acquisition cause a broad variability in the appearance of the objects. Generalization about the objects can not be done at hand rather each case that appears in practice should be stored into the system and the system should learn more generalized description for the different appearances of the same objects over time. All that suggests to take a case-based reasoning approach for the image interpretation rather than a generalized approach.

In this paper we present our strategy on building the intelligent image analysis and interpretation unit based on case-based reasoning. In Section 2 we give general comments to the image analysis of microorganism. Related work will be described in Section 3. The development issues are worked out in Section 4. Section 5 describes the fungal cultures and the image properties of the fungi spores. The developed image acquisition unit is described in Section 6. Section 7 shows how a case is represented. The architecture of the system is presented in Section 8. Finally we give results in Section 9.

## 2 General Comments to the Image Analysis of Microorganism

Classification of airborne fungal spores from environmental samples presents the image analyst with its own inherent difficulties. Most of these difficulties apply to the automatic identification of microorganism in general [2]. For example, the types and numbers of objects (different fungal species) that may be present in any one sample of the air are both unknown and effectively unlimited. Also, intra-species variation of characteristics (such as size, color or texture of spores) can be large, and dependent on several factor. Furthermore, the bulk size of two targeted species may be an order of magnitude or more apart, making decisions such as optical magnification setting a difficult choice. The dynamic and variable nature of the microorganism thus creates a formidable challenge to the design of a robust image interpretation system with the ideal characteristics of high analysis accuracy but with wide generalization ability. The difficulties can be summarized as follow:

- **Intra-species variation due to natural phenomenon, i.e., life-cycle, environmental effects**
  The dynamic nature of living organisms results in properties such as size, or color of the microorganism being statistically non-stationary. Different growth condition of microorganism may result in uncharacteristically large or small specimens – resulting in data outliners. Ultimately, the classification accuracy of an image interpretation system under these circumstances will rely on the training database capturing as much of this variability as possible.
- **Intra-species variation due to predation, fragmentation etc.**
  Often atypical characteristics occur due to predation, environmental factors, or aging.
- **To stain or not to stain?**
  Many species appear clear/opaque at the resolutions used, making imaging and analysis very difficult. Staining can help to increase the resolution of the fungal material and to distinguish between viable and non-viable organisms. Depending on the application different stains have to be used. At present 10-20 different stains are frequent used for staining fungal spores. There are "all-purpose"-stains such as lactophenol cotton blue which stains fungal elements blue. The staining procedure takes only 1 to 2 minutes. The application of fluorescence stains allows to discriminate between live and dead cells. However the use of epifluorescence microscopy in an automated system is more expensive and requires additional hardware. While it is common to stain specimen samples prior to analysis, staining puts special requirements to an automated probe handling, image acquisition system and image interpretation system.
- **Choosing an appropriate optical resolution for imaging specimens**
  The wide variation of the size of targeted species necessitates a choice of optical magnification that may not be optimal for any species. For example, to analyse the fine internal structures of species such as Wallemia sebi, a 1000x magnification would be required. Fusarium spores are the largest spores among the spores considered in this study. They would only require a 200x magnification instead of a 1000x magnification.
- **Imaging 3-dimensional objects**
  The spore is a 3-dimensional object. Imagine a spore which has an ellipsoid shape. Depending on the pose the object can appear as a round object or as a long elongated object in a 2-D image. Many species have a significant length in the third dimension - often greater than the depth-of-field of the imaging device - making their representation as a 2-D image is difficult. As such, significant areas of the specimen will be out of focus. If only one kind of specimen appears in an image to focus may not be so difficult. However, in a real air sample, different specimen can appear. Then one focus level may not be sufficient. Different levels of focus may be necessary which will result in more than one digital image for one probe.
- How to get a clean probe from the air sample?
  Samples of bioaerosols will contain a wide range of objects (organic and inorganic particles). Filters will be needed to remove particles larger than the objects of interest. But this will not prevent the image from non-targeted species in general. Non-targeted species/objects will generally need to be classified. Normally the probe should be covered by water and a cover glass. To realize this in an automated

handling system is not easy since handling devices are not good when handling class.

# 3 Related Work

There have been done several case studies on identifying fungi or other microorganism. In [3] is described an image analysis method for the identification of colonies of nine different Penicillium species as seen after growth on a standard medium. In [4] is described a study of image analysis based on fluorescence microscopy images for the improvement of the exposure assessment of airborne microorganism. Semiautomatic image analysis techniques are applied to segment the contour of fungal hyphae in [5]. Yeast cells are analyzed by image analysis techniques in [6]. Different *Fusarium* species macroconidia are analyzed in [7]. The work aims at designing an automated procedure for collecting and documenting microscopic pictures of *Fusarium* conidia, determining various morphological parameters and statistically evaluating the power of those characteristics in differentiating the most important pathogenic *Fusarium* species occurring on wheat in Germany.

The work which is most closely related to our work is the work described in [8]. The ability of an image analysis routine to differentiate between spores of eleven allergenic fungal genera was tested using image analysis based on seven basic and up to 17 more complex features, extracted from digitized images. Fungal spores of Alternaria, Cladosporium, Fusarium, Aspergillus, Botrytis, Penicillium, Epicoccum, Exserohilum, Ustilago, Coprinus and Psilocybe were examined in a series of experiments designed to differentiate between spores at the genus and species level. There is no specific algorithm for image enhancement and image segmentation described in this work. It seems that only the feature measurement has been automated. The object area was labelled interactively. From the fungal spores were extracted 7 basic features such as length, width, width/length ratio, area, form factor (circularity), perimeter and roundness and 17 more complex features; equivalent circular diameter, compactness, box area, radius, modification ratio, sphericity, convex hull area, convex hull perimeter, solidity, concavity, convexity, fibre length, fibre width. Linear and Quadratic discriminant analysis were used for classification. It is interesting to note that they have been created a sufficient large enough database of fungi spores for their analysis. The number of spores used for this study ranges from 200 to 1000 samples. The classification accuracy according to a particular class ranges from 56% to 93% for genera comparison and from 26% to 97% for species comparison. The results shows that not for all classes have been chosen the right features for classification. It rather seems that all common features that are known in pattern recognition for the description of a 2 D objects are applied to the images. There have not been developed specific features that describe the properties of the different fungi genera and species. To give an example what is meant consider specie Fusarium. In case of Fusarium is the septation a highly discriminating features but no such description is included in the feature list.

Finally, we can say there has been done a number of successfully case studies to automate the identification of fungi and in general microorganism. In these work there has been developed or applied imaging method for microorganism, automatic focussing methods, image analysis, feature description and classification. Most of these work use for the image acquisition 500x to 1500x magnification. The most used feature descriptors are the area size and the shape factor circularity. Only in case of [3] they use the color information. In all other work the color information is neglect. Not all work included microscopic images of the microorganism in the paper therefore we can not evaluate the quality of the images. Especially, for the identification of fungal spores in [7] and [8] we would have liked to see the images. In most of the cases the digitized images are not highly structured. The objects and the background appear more or less homogenous which allows to apply a simple thresholding technique for image segmentation. In general we an say that these work are characterized by applying standard image analysis and feature extraction procedures to the images. There has not been developed a specific feature set for fungi identification nor has been found a good feature set for the description of microorganism yet as it can be seen from [7] and [8].

The difference to our work is that in most of these studies are created images for only one specie and not for a variety of different species, except for the work in [8]. The creation of digitized images for a variety of different species is much harder since the species differ in size and dimension and, therefore, is the selection of an optical resolution which will show the images details of the different species in sufficient enough resolution not easy. Also, the image analysis is much more difficult since for all the different objects a sufficient image quality should be reached after image segmentation.

## 4 Development Issues

We decided to start the development of our system based on a data set of fungi spore images taken in the laboratory under optimal conditions and constant climate conditions. The data set should represent the prototypical appearance of the different kind of fungi strains and serve as gold standard. An image acquisition unit for the laboratory image acquisition was developed (see Section   ). Based on that equipment we are constantly collecting digital images of fungi spores grown under clear defined laboratory condition. At the end we will have a large enough image data set which can serve as the basis for our system development.

The objects in the images are good representatives of the different kinds of fungal spores cultured under optimal conditions and constant climate conditions. However, as it can be seen from the images of Alternaria alternata and Ulocladium botrytis none of the objects in the image looks like the other ones. There is no clear prototypical object. We can see a high biological variability and besides that we see younger and older representatives of the fungal strains. Depending on the image acquisition conditions we see objects from the side and top view that influences the appearance of the objects. Generalization about the objects can not be done at hand rather each case that appears in practice should be stored into the system and the system should learn more generalized description for the different appearance of the same objects over time. All that suggests to take a case-based reasoning approach for the image interpretation [9] rather than a generalized approach. Case-Based Reasoning [10] is used when generalized knowledge is lacking. The method works on a set of cases formerly processed and stored in a case base. A new case is interpreted by searching for similar cases in the case base. Among this set of similar cases the closest case with its associated result is selected and presented to the output.

For the kind of images created in the laboratory we have to develop an image analysis procedure. Then we need to describe the images by image features and to develop a feature extraction procedure which can automatically extract the features from the images. The features and the feature values extracted from the images together with the name of the fungal spores make up an initial description of the data. We do not know if all image features are necessary. However we extract as much as possible image features from the images which make sense in some way to ensure that we can mine the right case description from this database. From this initial description of the data we need to identify good representative descriptions for the cases by using case mining methods [10]. Based on that information we will built up the case-based reasoning system.

After we have reached a sufficient enough classification accuracy we will go over to include real air samples into the system by adapting the prototypical representations of fungi spores to the real ones. However, at the moment we are fair from this step.

## 5 Fungal Cultures and Property Description

Six fungal strains representing species with different spore types were used for the study (Tab. 1). The strains were obtained from the fungal stock collection of the Institute of Microbiology, University of Jena/ Germany and from culture collection of JenaBios GmbH. All strains were cultured in Petri dishes on 2 % maltextract agar (Merck) at 24°C in an incubation chamber for at least 14 days. For microscopy fungal spores were scrapped off from the agar surface and placed on a microscopic slide in a drop of lactic acid. Naturally hyaline spores were additional stained with lactophenol cotton blue (Merck). A database of images from the spores of these species were produced. The number of imaged spore per specie was about 30-50.

## 6 Image Acquisition

Image acquisition were conducted using a Zeiss-Axiolab transmission light microscope equipped with a 100x lens and a NIKON Coolpix 4500 digital color camera. The magnification is 1000x using a 100x objective. The resulting pixel size ranges from 0,1 to 0,025 μm. The average spore size of common airborne fungi varies between 2 to 40 μm. Some digitized sample images are presented in Figure 1 for the different fungal spores. The objects in the images are good representatives of the different kinds of fungal spores cultured under optimal conditions and constant climate conditions.

**Table 1.** Strains of fungi used and selected properties of spores

| Species | Strain - no.* | Spore shape** | Spore color** | Spore size (µm)** |
|---|---|---|---|---|
| Alternaria alternata | J 37 (B) | Septated, clavate to ellipsoid | Pale brown | 18-83 x 7-18 |
| Aspergillus niger | i400 (A) | Spherical, ornamented with warts and spines | Brown | 3,5 - 5 in diam. |
| Rhizopus stolonifer | J 07 (B) | Irregular in shape, often ovoid to elliptical, striate | Pale brown | 7-15 x 6-8 |
| Scopulariopsis brevicaulis | J26 (B) | Spherical to ovoid | Rose-brown | 5-8 x 5-7 |
| Ulocladium botrytis | i171(A) | Septated, ellipsoid | Olive-brown | 18-38 x 11-20 |
| Wallemia sebi | J 35 (B) | Cubic to globose | Pale-brown | 2,5 - 3,5 in diam. |

*: (A) from the fungal stock collection of the Institute of Microbiology, University of Jena/ Germany
*: (B) from culture collection of JenaBios GmbH/ Germany
**: adapted from [11]

## 7 Case Description

An image may be described by the pixel matrix itself or by parts of this matrix (a pixel representation) [12]. It may be described by the objects contained in the image and their features (a feature-based representation) [13]. Furthermore, it can be described by a more complex model of the image scene comprising objects and their features as well as the object's spatial relationships (an attributed graph representation [14] or semantic network [15]).

We choose an attribute-value pair representation for the case description. The case consists of the solution which is the type of fungi spores and the features describing the visual properties of the object (see Figure 2). The features are color, shape, special properties inside the objects such as structure inside, size, and appearance of the cell contour.

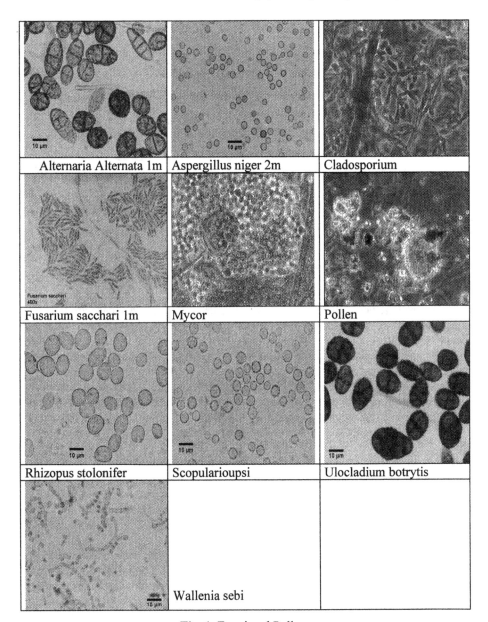

**Fig. 1.** Fungi and Pollen

Description
Color = brown
Object= is structured
Contour=double contour
Shape=bottle-like shapes

Solution
**Alternaria Alternata**

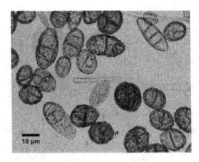

**Fig. 2.** Example of a Case Description

## 8 The Architecture

The recent architecture of the system is shown in Figure 3.

The cases are image descriptions which are automatically extracted from the images based on the procedures installed in the feature extraction unit and stored into the case base together with the class name. In a separate image database are kept all images, class names, and image descriptions given by an human operator for later evaluation purposes.

Image analysis is done by transforming the color image into a gray-level image, the image smoothing, and a shape-based matching procedure for object recognition.

The feature extraction unit contains feature extraction procedures that have been identified based on the interview with the expert. We should note here that a particular application requires special feature descriptors. Therefore not all possible feature extraction procedure can be implemented into such a system from scratch. But we hope that we can come up with a special vocabulary and the associated feature extraction procedures for our application on fungi identification.

Similarity between an actual case and cases in case base should be determined based on the Euclidean distance. The initial case base is a flat case base. An index structure and more compact case description are incrementally learnt as soon as new cases are input into the case base. For that we will use decision tree learning and prototype learning methods [16].

The case base maintenance process will start when the expert criticizes the result of the system. In that case the wrong fungi species has be identified by the system. Then it has to be checked by the system developer whether new features have to be acquired for each case or the case representation should be updated based on the learning procedures. To acquire new features means that the necessary feature extraction procedures have to be developed and for all cases in the case base the new features have to be calculated and inputted into the existing case description. Then the case representation has to be updated as well as the index structure. However, this ensures that we can come up step-by-step with a system which can describe the variability of the different biological objects that can appear in real life.

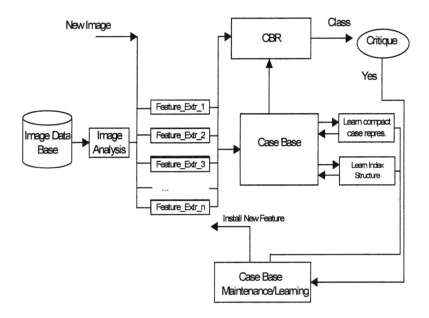

**Fig. 3.** Architecture of the System

## 9 Recent Results

The image acquisition unit was developed (see Section  ) and a data base of 10 up to 20 images for each kind of specie containing 30-50 spores was recently collected.

The original color image is transformed to a grey level image by using the following formula:  $grey = 0.299 * red + 0.587 * green + 0.144 * blue$ . The image is filtered by a Gauss filter in order to reduce noise. Afterwards image equalization is applied in order to reduce illumination effects.

Since the different fungi spores have a shape that will be relatively constant independent from the life-cycle effect we use a shape-based matching procedure [17] in order to recognize objects in the image. Two different shape models have been created, one for a circle and one for a ellipse, see Figure 4. The figure shows sample images for two different kind of fungi spores and the results obtained by the matching procedure. The shapes of the different fungi species can be covered by these models. The shapes of the fungi vary in scale and illumination. They can be occluded and clutter. The model consists of a set of points and their corresponding direction vectors. In the matching process, a transformed model is compared to the image at a particular location by a similarity measure. The normalized dot product of the direction vectors of the transformed model and the search image over all points of the model is used to compute a matching score at a particular point of the image. The normalized similarity measure has the property that it returns a number smaller than 1 as the score of a potential match. A score of 1 indicates a perfect match between the model and the image. Furthermore, the score roughly corresponds to the portion of the model that is visible in the image. Once the object has been recognized on the lowest level of the image pyramid, its position, rotation, and scale are extracted to a resolution better than the discretization of the search space by fitting the second order polynomial (in the four pose variables horizontal translation, vertical translation, rotation, and scale) to the similarity measure values in a 3 x 3 x 3 x 3 neighborhood around the maximum score.

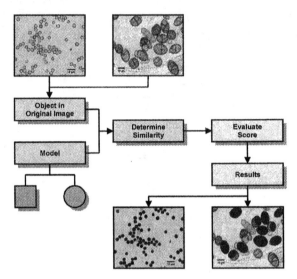

**Fig. 4.** Object Recognition

## 10 Conclusion

We have described our recent results on the development of an image interpretation system  for the identification of airborne fungi. Such a system is important for the continuous registration of biological working substances which have an influence to human health. The paper gives general comments to the image analysis of microorganism. The resulting development issues have a high influence to methods which can be applied in the system and to the system architecture. The fungal culture and the image properties of the fungi spores are described. Based on an image acquisition system for the laboratory we create an digital image data base from the fungi spores. That gives us the basis for the development of the image interpretation system. Features that describe the objects could be identified based on an expert interview and make up the initial case description. Since it is not clear how relevant and discriminative the features are the case base maintenance process has also to include the identification and installation of new feature extraction procedures. Besides that a representative case description and the index structure over the case base should be learnt incrementally. Finally, we showed first results on the image analysis. Shape-based matching can be used for the recognition of the objects.

The described solution is the intelligent heart of the complete system for the automatic registration of airborne fungi. The complete system will comprise a handling unit, an image acquisition unit, and the intelligent image interpretation unit.

## Acknowledgement

The project "Development of methods and techniques for the image-acquisition and computer-aided analysis of biologically dangerous substances BIOGEFA" is sponsored by the German Ministry of Economy BMWI under the grant number 16IN0147.

## References

1. F.H.L. Benyon, A.S. Jones, E.R. Tovey and G. Stone, Differentiation of allergenic fungal spores by image analysis, with application to aerobiological counts, Aerobiologia 15: 211-223, 1999
2. R.F. Walker and M. Kumagai, Image Analysis as a Tool for Quantitative Phycology – A Computational Approach to Cyanobacterial Taxa Identification, Limnology, vol. 1, No. 2, pp. 107-115
3. Th. Dörge, J.M. Carstensen, J. Ch. Frisvad, Direct Identification of pure Penicillium species using image analysis, Journal of Microbiological Methods 41(2000), 121-133
4. J. Kildesø, B.H. Nielsen, Exposure Assesment of Airborne Microorganisms by Fluorescence Microscopy and Image Processing, Annual Occupational Hygiene, vol. 41, No. 2, pp. 201-216, 1997
5. Inglis IM and Gray AJ 2001: An evaluation of semiautomatic approaches to contour segmentation applied to fungal hyphae. Biometrics 57(1), 232-239.
6. M.-N. Pons, H. Vivier, Morphometry of Yeast, In: M.H.F. Wilkinson and F. Schut (Eds.), Digital Image Analysis of Microbes: Imaging, Morphometry, Fluorometry and Motility Techniques and Applications, John Wiley & Sons Ltd., 1998
7. S. Gottwald, Ch. U. Germeier, W. Ruhmann, Computerized image analysis in Fusarium taxonomy, Mycol. Research, 105 (2), p. 206-214.
8. F.H.L. Benyon, A.S. Jones, E.R. Tovey and G. Stone, Differentiation of allergenic fungal spores by image analysis, with application to aerobiological counts, Aerobiologia 15: 211-223, 1999
9. P. Perner, Why Case-Based Reasoning is Attractive for Image Interpretation, International Conference on Case-Based Reasoning, ICCBR2001, Vancouver Canada, In: D. Aha and I. Watson (Eds.), Case-Bases Reasoning Research and Developments, Springer Verlag 2001, lnai 2080, p. 27-44.
10. P. Perner, Data Mining on Multimedia Data, Springer Verlag 2003
11. R. Samson, E.S. Hoekstra, J.C. Frisvad, O. Filtenborg (Eds.), Indroduction to food-and airborne fungi, Centraalbureau voor Schimmelcultures
12. P. Perner, An Architeture for a CBR Image Segmentation System, Journal on Engineering Application in Artificial Intelligence, Engineering Applications of Artificial Intelligence, vol. 12 (6), 1999, p. 749-759

13. P. Perner,H. Perner, and B. Müller, Similarity Guided Improvement of the System Performance in an Image Classification System, In: S. Craw and A.Preece (Eds.), Advances in Case-Based Reasoning, ECCBR2002, Springer Verlag, lnai 2416, 2002, p. 604-612.
14. Grimnes, M. & Aamodt, A.(1996). A two layer case-based reasoning architecture for medical image understanding, In I. Smith & B. Faltings (Eds.) *Advances in Case-Based Reasoning* (pp. 164-178). Berlin: Springer Verlag.
15. Perner, P. (1998). Using CBR learning for the low-level and high-level unit of a image interpretation system. In S. Singh (Ed.) *Advances in Pattern Recognition* (pp. 45-54). Berlin: Springer Verlag.
16. A. Aamodt, H.A. Sandtorv, O.M. Winnem, Combining Case-Based Reasoning and Data Mining – A Way of Revealing and Reusing RAMS Experience, Lydersen, Hansen and Sandorv (Eds.): Safety and Reliability, Proc. of ESREL`98, Trondheim, 1998, pp. 1345-1351.
17. Steger, C., Similarity measures for occlusion, clutter, and illumination invariant object recognition. In: B. Radig and S. Florczyk (Eds.), Mustererkennung 2001, Springer, München, pp. 148-154.

# Quantification and Characterization of Pulmonary Emphysema in Multislice-CT

## A Fully Automated Approach

Oliver Weinheimer[1,2], Tobias Achenbach[1], Christian Buschsiewke[1],
Claus Peter Heussel[1], Thomas Uthmann[2], and Hans-Ulrich Kauczor[3]

[1] Dept. of Radiology, Johannes Gutenberg-University of Mainz,
D-55101 Mainz, Germany
mail@oliwe.com, http://www.oliwe.com

[2] Inst. of Computer Science, Johannes Gutenberg-University, D-55099 Mainz

[3] DKFZ Dept. of Radiology, German Cancer Research Center, D-69120 Heidelberg

**Abstract.** The new technology of the Multislice-CT provides volume data sets with approximately isotropic resolution, which permits a non invasive measurement of diffuse lung diseases like emphysema in the 3D space. The aim of our project is the development of a full automatic 3D CAD (Computer Aided Diagnosis) software tool for detection, quantification and characterization of emphysema in a thoracic CT data set. It should supply independently an analysis of an image data set to support the physician in clinical daily routine. In this paper we describe the developed 3D algorithms for the segmentation of the tracheo-bronchial tree, the lungs and the emphysema regions. We present different emphysema describing indices.

## 1  Introduction

On CT images of emphysema patients an abnormal, permanent enlargement of the air spaces distal to the terminal bronchioles accompanied by destruction of the bronchiolar walls can be registered. The classical method of CT image evaluation is the pixel index (PI). It was introduced by Kalender et al. [KR1]. The PI is the percentage of voxels in the lung with a smaller CT value than a limit value. Blechschmidt et al. [BW1] presented an algorithm of thoracic CT image evaluation based on 2D morphology of emphysema.

Our CT image evaluation is based on 3D morphology of emphysema. The procedure of the fully automated 3D CAD tool can be divided roughly into the following 3 steps:

1. Searching of landmarks in a CT volume
2. Reconstruction of the lungs and the tracheo-bronchial tree
3. Detection, quantification and characterization of emphysema

Due to the limited space available, the individual steps are only briefly described in the sections 2, 3 and 4. Finally, a presentation of the results in patient data sets and a perspective of the project is given.

P. Perner et al. (Eds.): ISMDA 2003, LNCS 2868, pp. 75–82, 2003.

We used thoracic Multislice-CT images in the DICOM format from a Siemens Multislice-CT scanner (Volume Zoom, Siemens Medical Engineering Group, Erlangen, Germany). The voxelsize varied between $0.5 \times 0.5 \times 1.25 \, mm^3$ and $0.8 \times 0.8 \times 1.25 \, mm^3$, with a slice increment of $1{,}0 \, mm$.

## 2    Searching of Landmarks

In order to reconstruct the tracheo-bronchial tree and the lungs several landmarks are searched within the trachea, the right and the left lung, which permit as starting points a reconstruction of these structures. All found landmarks are held in a list and can be edited manually over a landmark administration window.

The trachea search e. g. is realized on the "upper slices"[4] of a data set. A body detection is performed, so that the search area for the trachea can be limited to the body region. Fig. 1(a) shows the sequence of the body detection.

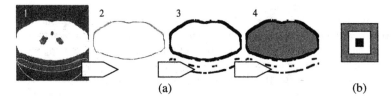

(a)                                                        (b)

**Fig. 1.** (a) The different stages of body detection. 1. Original image. 2. Body edge voxel marked. 3. After dilatation on body edge voxels with a 5x5 window as structue element. 4. After region growing within body edge voxels started at the image center. The body region is marked grey. (b) Mask for trachea search within in the body.

In order to identify a trachea landmark the mask as shown in fig. 1(b) is used. In a 5x5-window around a voxel it is examined whether the average HU value is <-975 HU (black window in fig.1(b), definitely air). In a "perforated" neighborhood (grey range in fig. 1(b)) it is examined, whether all voxels are above -525 HU (tissue, definitely not air). If both conditions are fulfilled, a simple threshold based 2D region growing (threshold -800 HU) is started. If the growing results in an area smaller than $8 \, cm^2$ [5], the initially voxel is used as trachea landmark, otherwise the search will be continued. The algorithm stops, if a trachea point is found, or if no suitable trachea point could be identified on 20 neighbouring slices.

---

[4] The upper slices can be determined with the help of the tag "slice location" in the header of the DICOM-files.
[5] Because the maximal accepted trachea radius is smaller than $1.5 \, cm$.

# 3    Reconstructions of Lungs and Tracheo-Bronchial Tree

## 3.1    Tracheo-Bronchial Tree Tracer

In [CH1] a 2D procedure for finding and measuring bronchi in axial HRCT images is described and [MH1] presents a hybrid procedure, consisting of 2D and 3D modules, for segmenting the tracheo-bronchial tree. We introduce a pure 3D algorithm motivated by these procedures.

The automatic landmark search supplies a starting point for the bronchial tree tracer within the trachea (see section 2). It can also be set manually if the search fails. On the basis of this starting point, a special region growing with a N26 neighbourhood system starts. Following growing conditions are used:

1. Mean value in N27 or N7 neighborhood <-950 HU (see fig. 2(a)(b)).
2. no value >-800 HU in N27 .

If the conditions are fulfilled, a voxel is marked as "bronchusL" (L for large). The conditions are selected so restrictively that "leaking out" of the segmentation into the lung parenchyma is not possible.

If the conditions are not fulfilled, it is examined whether the voxel is in a smaller bronchus. The rationale of the 2nd, more difficult, evaluation is the following: a bronchus will be truncated either in the axial, coronal or sagittal plane in a circularly to elliptically way (see fig. 2(c)(d)). If a voxel lies within a bronchus, then it is surrounded by bronchial wall in one of the planes in all directions. The algorithm does not examine all directions, but in each plane 8 rays as direction of detection are casted outward (see fig. 2(e)(f)).

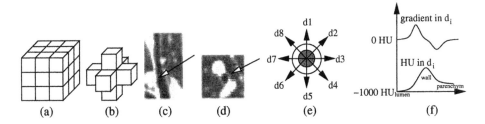

(a)     (b)     (c)     (d)     (e)     (f)

**Fig. 2.** (a) N27 corresponds to a cube with side length 3. (b) N7-window. In these two structure elements the HU values are examined. (c) A bronchus in the axial view. (d) Same bronchus in the coronal view as a round cut. (e) Schematic representation of a bronchus. Each bronchus is either in the sagittal, coronal or axial plane cut in a circularly or elliptically way. Since the bronchi have a small diameter, it is sufficient casting out rays in the 8 drawn directions. (f) Profile of gradient and of HU values in direction $d_i$.

On each ray the maximal positive gradient $(grad_i)_{1 \leq i \leq 8}$ and the maximal HU value $(max_i)_{1 \leq i \leq 8}$ are determined. In order to decide whether or not a voxel belongs to the bronchial tree for each plane a procedure similar to the discrete ERS transform introduced in [CH1] is done. In a nutshell, it is determined if a voxel is air and if it is surrounded by airway wall in one plane in all directions. Again the conditions are selected so restrictively that "leaking out" into the lung parenchyma is not possible.

If a voxel is identified as lumen voxel in one plane, the voxel is marked according to the plane in which it has been identified as "bronchusS" (sagittal), "bronchusC" (coronal) or "bronchusA" (axial). Fig. 3 shows a bronchial tree segmented with this procedure.

## 3.2   Lung Tissue Reconstruction

On the basis of starting points in both lungs (see section 2), the lung parenchyma is first marked as lung with a simple threshold based region growing and a N6 (3D) neighborhood system (threshold -500 HU[6]). In the next step only the voxels marked as lung are considered. We handle the lung segmentation like a stack of binary images. The goal is marking areas as lung, which lie in the lung, but were not marked as lung by the threshold based region growing (e.g. lung vessels). This is reached by two morphological steps in the axial images:

1. Dilatation of the segmentation lung with a 3x3-window as structure element.
2. Filling of holes, whereby a hole is defined as a set of not marked lung voxels which are not connected with the image border (see [S1]).

Fig. 3(c) shows results of the lung tissue reconstruction.

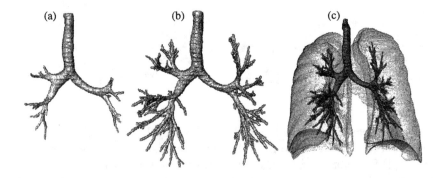

**Fig. 3.** (a) Visualization of voxels marked as "BronchusL". (b) Final result of the bronchial tree segmentation. (c) Bronchial tree with the segmented lung tissue.

---

[6] For lung tissue reconstruction in literature often values between -200 and -500 HU are used (see e. g. [BW1]).

## 4    Detection, Quantification, and Characterization of Emphysema

The emphysema analyzing algorithm needs a segmented tracheo-bronchial tree and a lung segmentation as precondition. First voxels with a density <-950 HU (air), which corresponds to the lung but not to the tracheo-bronchial tree, are marked as emphysema voxels.

Subsequently, an error correction of the segmentation is realized: Therefore all voxels, below a threshold of -910 HU and which are surrounded by emphysema voxels are also marked as emphysema in order to correct the partial volume effect and image noise. In a third step the emphysema is characterized[7]:

1. The distance of emphysema voxels to lung pleura is measured. If distance <20 $mm$, emphysema voxels are marked as peripheral.
2. All emphysema voxels are divided in border and inner voxels. An emphysema voxel is an inner voxel, if in its N4 (2D) neighborhood all voxel are marked as emphysema.
3. An emphysema voxel is considered as "panlobular", if the distance to a non-emphysema voxel is greater than 2 $mm$.

Afterall, a determination of contiguous emphysema regions (low attenuation areas, cluster) is performed by repeated region growing. The total volume data set is passed through sequentially. If the algorithm detects an emphysema voxel, which does not belong to a cluster, a region growing starts. Emphysema voxels are added to the cluster, if in the N8 (2D) neighborhood 4 further emphysema voxel occur. For the growing of the emphysema cluster, a divided neighbourhood system is used[8]:

1. If the voxel, that is just added to the current cluster, is *not* "panlobular", then the N4 (2D) neighbourhood system is used ⇒ 2D growing.
2. If the voxel, that is just added to the current cluster, is "panlobular", then the N6 (3D) neighbourhood system is used ⇒ 3D growing.

The clusters are divided in size classes according to Blechschmidt et al. [BW1], who only used 2D clusters. Four cluster sizes are identified[9]: class 0: $\geq 2$ $mm^3$, class 1: $\geq 8$ $mm^3$ , class 2: $\geq 65$ $mm^3$ class 3: $\geq 120$ $mm^3$. Single emphysema cluster are held in a list and can be shown at the screen by click (e.g for planning local surgery).

The following, emphysema describing indices, are calculated:

1. Mean lung density (MLD) in HU.
2. Emphysema index (EI or PI): $(|emphysema\,voxel|/|lung\,voxel|) * 100$, i.e. how much per cent lung belongs to emphysema.

---

[7] The size of a secondary lobulus is between 5 $mm$ and 20 $mm$. An emphysema region is called panlobular, if a whole secondary lobulus is destroyed. Smaller emphysema regions are called centrilobular. A peripheral lying panlobular emphysema region is called paraseptal (more precise definitions e.g. in [BR1]).

[8] Because the x,y-resolution is higher than the z-resolution.

[9] The standard values for the four 3D cluster sizes are calculated with the sphere formular $4 * \Pi * r^3/3$. The values for r are taken from Blechschmidt et al. [BW1].

3. Bullae index (BI):

$$BI = \frac{\sum_{i=0}^{3} w_{class\,i} * g_{class\,i}}{\sum_{i=0}^{3} w_{class\,i} * 4} * 10 \text{ with } w_{class\,i} \text{ for the weight of class i,}$$

$$p_{class\,i} = \frac{|emphysema\ voxel\ in\ class_i|}{|lung\ voxel|} * 100$$

$$\text{and } g_{class\,i} = \begin{cases} p_{class\,i}, & if\ 0 \le p_{class\,i} \le 4 \\ 4, & if\ p_{class\,i} \ge 4 \end{cases}.$$

The weights of the classes are given by standard with 1,2,3 and 4 , i.e. voxels in $class_3$ opposite a voxels in $class_0$ rates quadruple. So BI ranges from zero to ten, BI of 0 means no emphysema and an BI of 10 means a lot of emphysema cluster in all size classes.

4. $ET1 =(|inner\ voxel| / |border\ voxel|) * 10$. The greater this value, the larger the emphysema clusters.

5. $ET2 =(|peripheral\ voxel| / |emphysema\ voxel|)*100$. The greater this value, the more predominant is the localization in the subpleural space.

6. $ET3 =(|panlobular\ voxel| / |emphysema\ voxel|) * 100$. Similar to ET1, but this index provides first indications only if whole lobules are destroyed.

Note the fact, that single emphysema voxels lie below the smallest cluster size and thus they are not considered in the computation of the bullae index, what can be interpreted as an additional noise correction. All parameters of the algorithm are selectable (e. g. cluster sizes, clusterweights, thresholds).

## 5   Experimental Results

A preliminary analysis of the emphysema tool was carried out using 15 data sets acquired in patients with and without emphysema. Searching of the landmarks in the trachea and in the lungs was successful in all data sets. The segmentations of the bronchial tree and the lung was accomplished with all patients. The bronchial tree tracer ran stable and detected partly bronchi up to the 8. generation. Tab. 1 shows results of the CAD tool.

Due to different pathologies of emphysema (e.g. centrilobular and panlobular) a single emphysema index is not able to describe emphysema in all cases. The consultation of different indices is used to compensate this. Note, that for all normal patients $(n)$ of tab. 1 $BI < 1$, $ET1 < 3$ and $ET3 \approx 0$, for patients with centrilobular emphysema $(c)$ $BI > 1$, $ET1 > 3$ and $ET3 > 0$, and for patients with strong panlobular emphysema $(p^+ - p^{++})$ $ET3 >> 0$.

E.g. patient #14 of tab. 1: an EI of 10.5 is in a range, that does not indicate of emphysema. Also a MLD of -810 HU is a normal value. In contrast an increased BI (4.9) and strongly increased values for ET1 (24.8) and ET3 (36.7) are registered. Fig. 4 shows images of this emphysema patient, who has large emphysema bullae in the upper lobes. This demonstrates that a set of 3 indices (BI, ET1 and ET3) provides a suitable description of emphysema extent and form. This will be addressed in detailed in a larger clinical study.

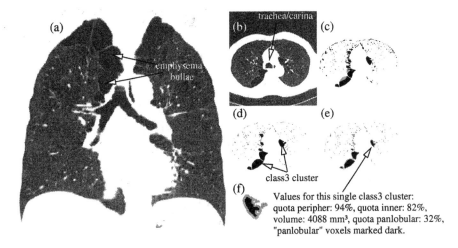

**Fig. 4.** (a) Coronal image of patient #14 (see tab. 1). Emphysema bullae in the upper lung regions (see arrow). (b) Axial image of same patient. (c) Peripheral emphysema voxels marked dark, not peripheral ones light gray. (d) Emphysema cluster of $class_3$ are marked in dark, smaller cluster are marked in light grey. Note, that the parts of the bronchial tree are excluded. (e) "Panlobular" voxels marked dark, not "panlobular" voxels light gray. (f) One single selected $class_3$ cluster and its describing values. ⇒ The cluster is peripher and panlobular. ⇒ It is a *paraseptal* emphysema cluster.

## 6   Perspective

The segmentation of the tracheo-bronchial tree will be transferred into a skeletonization (see [PS1, M1]). From this skeleton a graph representation of the trachea-bronchial tree will be derived, whereby the nodes of the graph correspond to the branchpoints of the skeleton representation. The nomenclature of the bronchi will be accomplished by an "attributed tree matching" procedure [PS2, KP1].

Subsequently, the labeled bronchi can be measured in 3D. Several lung diseases are associated with an increase of the airway wall thickness, its measurement could be a further important parameter.

With the help of the labeled bronchial tree and the visible fissures lung segmentation will be divided in lobes and segments. Then the emphysema clusters can be attributed to specific lobes or segments.

## References

[BW1]  R. A. Blechschmidt, R. Werthschützky, U. Lörcher: Automated CT Image Evaluation of the Lung: A Morphology-Based Concept. IEEE Transactions on medical imaging, vol. 20, no. 5, may 2001.

**Table 1.** Results of the emphysema tool. c = centrilobular emphysema, p = panlobular emphysema and n = normal. + refers to the severity of emphysema.

| patient # | trachea land-mark | lung land-mark | lung volume $mm^3$ | trachea volume $mm^3$ | EI % | BI | ET1 | ET2 % | ET3 % | MLD HU | visual radiological diagnosis |
|---|---|---|---|---|---|---|---|---|---|---|---|
| 1 | found | found | 7684 | 107 | 37 | 7.5 | 19.9 | 50.0 | 18.4 | -875 | $c^{++}$ / $p^{++}$ |
| 2 | found | found | 7339 | 113 | 16.8 | 6.5 | 4.5 | 52.5 | 1.9 | -858 | c |
| 3 | found | found | 5541 | 70 | 3.9 | 0.8 | 1.7 | 67.8 | 0.0 | -831 | n |
| 4 | found | found | 6622 | 111 | 17.5 | 7.0 | 5.9 | 51.3 | 0.6 | -851 | p |
| 5 | found | found | 4357 | 72 | 8.9 | 4.9 | 20.6 | 61.0 | 25.0 | -754 | $p^+$ |
| 6 | found | found | 7278 | 80 | 3.3 | 1.3 | 3.5 | 80.2 | 0.6 | -800 | c / p |
| 7 | found | found | 8383 | 118 | 22.7 | 7.9 | 4.2 | 48.9 | 0.3 | -864 | c |
| 8 | found | found | 3643 | 53 | 27.8 | 8.0 | 14.3 | 67.7 | 3.6 | -862 | c / p |
| 9 | found | found | 4525 | 109 | 0.8 | 0.1 | 1.8 | 75.6 | 0.0 | -765 | n |
| 10 | found | found | 5355 | 128 | 11.1 | 4.1 | 3.6 | 64.7 | 0.1 | -848 | c |
| 11 | found | found | 7484 | 109 | 11.1 | 6.3 | 7.2 | 66.1 | 1.5 | -830 | c / p |
| 12 | found | found | 3738 | 57 | 0.6 | 0.1 | 2.4 | 85.9 | 0.1 | -789 | n |
| 13 | found | found | 5034 | 83 | 3.3 | 0.8 | 2.1 | 62.4 | 0.1 | -806 | n |
| 14 | found | found | 6117 | 110 | 10.5 | 4.9 | 24.8 | 75.8 | 36.7 | -810 | c / $p^{++}$ |
| 15 | found | found | 5377 | 97 | 4.1 | 1.8 | 5.7 | 86.6 | 3.4 | -811 | c / p |

[BR1] R. C. Bittner, R. Roßdeutscher: Leitfaden Radiologie. Gustav Fischer Verlag, 1996

[CH1] F. Chabat, X.-P. Hu, D. M. Hansell, G.-Z Yang: ERS Transform for the Automated Detection of Bronchial Abnormalities on CT of the Lungs. IEEE Transactions on Medical Imaging, Vol. 20, No. 9, September 2001.

[KP1] H. Kitaoka, Y. Park, J. Tschirren, J. Reinhardt, M. Sonka, G. McLennan, E. A. Hoffmann: Automated Nomenclature Labeling of the Bronchial Tree in 3D-CT Lung Images. MICCAI 2002, LNCS 2489, pp. 1-11, 2002.

[KR1] W.A. Kalender, R. Rienmueller, W. Seissler, J. Behr, M. Welke, H. Fichte: Measurement of pulmonary parenchymal attenuation: use of spirometric gating with quantitative CT, Radiology, vol. 175, no. 1, pp. 265-268,1990

[M1] D. G. Morgenthaler: Three-Dimensional Simple Points: Serial Erosion, Parallel Thinning and Skeletonization. TR-1005, Computer Vision Laboratory, University of Maryland, 1981.

[MH1] D. Mayer, S. Ley, B.S. Brook, S. Thust, C.P. Heussel, H.-U. Kauczor: 3D-Segmentierung des menschlichen Trachiobronchialbaums aus CT-Bilddaten. Bildverarbeitung für die Medizin 2003, Springer Verlag, pp. 333-337, 2003

[PS1] K. Palagyi, E. Sorantin, E. Balogh, A. Kuba, C. Halmai, B. Erdöhelyi, K. Hausegger: A Sequential 3D Thinning Algorithm and its Medical Applications. IPMI 2001, LNCS 2082, pp. 409-415, 2001.

[PS2] M. Pelillo, K. Siddiqi, S. W. Zucker: Matching Hierarchical Structures Using Association Graphs. IEEE Transactions on Pattern Analysis and Machine Intelligence, Vol. 21, No. 11, November 1999.

[S1] P. Soille: Morphologische Bildverarbeitung. Springer-Verlag, 1998.

# Interactive Visualization of Diagnostic Data from Cardiac Images Using 3D Glyphs

Soo-Mi Choi[1], Don-Su Lee[1], Seong-Joon Yoo[1], Myoung-Hee Kim[2]

[1] Sejong University, School of Computer Engineering, 98 Gunja-dong, Gwangjin-gu,
Seoul 143-747, Korea
smchoi@sejong.ac.kr,
chunshanghwa@hanmail.net, sjyoo@sejong.ac.kr
[2] Ewha Womans University, Department of Computer Science and Engineering,
11-1 Daehyun-dong, Seodaemun-gu, Seoul 120-750, Korea
mhkim@ewha.ac.kr

**Abstract.** This paper describes accurate methods for measuring diagnostic data in cardiology and presents new ideas on interactive data visualization with 3D glyphs to get better insight about the measured data. First, we reconstruct the 3D shape and motion of the left ventricle from cardiac images using our time-varying deformable model. Then we accurately compute ventricular volume, mass, wall thickness and wall motion in 3D or 4D spaces. The computed data are interactively visualized in a qualitative and quantitative manner and can be combined into a single glyph. Thus, glyph-based interactive visualization can encode more information and can give access to several aspects of diagnostic data at once. This perceptually easy interface is useful for many diagnostic and patient monitoring applications.

## 1 Introduction

While many efforts have been made in the area of medical image visualization within the last decade, the visualization of diagnostic data extracted from the images has received much less attention. Data visualization is an emerging field whose goal is the perceptualization of information. A set of data usually includes some attributes or variables.

When diagnosing heart disease using 4D images, physicians typically have to estimate ventricular volume, ejection fraction, myocardial mass, wall motion, wall thickness and thickening, etc. They usually calculate ventricular volume by using several slice images with simplified equations and estimate ventricular motion by visual interpretation of wall motion in a cine loop. However, such methods are generally limited by assumptions about ventricular shape particularly when the ventricle is distorted by myocardial infarction. And the mental reconstruction of ventricular motion doesn't always give the same results at a regional level.

P. Perner et al. (Eds.): ISMDA 2003, LNCS 2868, pp. 83–90, 2003.
© Springer-Verlag Berlin Heidelberg 2003

Pentland *et al.* [1] used deformation modes to recover the non-rigid motion and structure of the left ventricle (LV) from X-ray images. Chen *et al.* [2] developed a hierarchical motion model by combining several existing simple models. Chen presented a scheme for left ventricular shape and motion modeling, analysis and visualization using angiographic data. McInerney and Terzopoulos [3] developed a dynamic finite element surface model for left ventricular segmentation, reconstruction and tracking. Nastar and Ayache [4] proposed a complex non-rigid deformation model of the LV only by a few parameters: the main excited modes and the main Fourier harmonics. Park *et al.* [5] developed a volumetric deformable model for the analysis of left ventricular motion from MRI-SPAMM in which some sparse points are produced to help the process of tracking. Bardinet *et al.* [6] proposed a parametric deformable model based on a superquadric fit followed by free form deformation.

Although previous approaches give satisfying results in the aspects of shape and motion visualization of the LV, it is not easy to get clinically useful information from cardiac images because of complicated pre- and/or post-processing. Another limitation occurs when 2D techniques are routinely used to estimate some diagnostic data that should be clarified in 3D or 4D spaces. Besides, data visualization in medical areas usually emphasizes the display of raw data and doesn't focus on the issue of interactive visualization associated with perceptual elements. In our previous work, we developed a new deformation model to represent the shape and motion of the LV of the heart [7,8]. This paper presents accurate methods for measuring clinically useful data based on the model including the validation of the methods and gives new ideas on interactive visualization with 3D glyphs for cardiac diagnosis.

This paper is organized as follows: Section 2 shortly describes our previous modeling framework and Section 3 describes the measurement of diagnostic data in 3D or 4D spaces for the analysis of ventricular function. Section 4 presents the visualization of diagnostic data using 3D glyphs. Finally, some conclusions are given in Section 5.

## 2   Reconstructing the Shape and Motion of the LV from Images

The developed deformation model [7,8] for the LV is based on three key ideas described as follows: First, a body-centered moving coordinate system is computed at each time step using natural vibration modes. The positions of points in the model are uniquely determined by how they are positioned within each vibration mode that corresponds to the object's generalized axes of symmetry. The coordinate system facilitates the tracking of the non-rigid motion of endo- and epicardial walls of the LV. Second, the process of cardiac deformation is considered to be a continuous function of material properties and virtual forces acting on the walls. Therefore, finite element method and modal analysis are used to compute numerical approximations. The required computational time is significantly reduced without loss of accuracy by ordering natural modes in terms of frequency of vibration and discarding high-frequency modes. Moreover, the reconstructed shapes are relatively robust for disambiguate input data because of the stability of low-frequency modes. Third, an interpolation function based on a 3D Gaussian function is used to create a model derived from input image and a new blob-like 3D finite element is formulated for the interpolation function. Unlike the existing methods based on a prototype, it calculates deformation modes directly from available image data. As a result, more improved natural shape parameterization was obtained. We applied the developed model to a patient with ischemic heart disease and a patient with coronary heart disease. Fig. 1 shows 3D reconstruction of endo- and epicardial walls at two key frames in the cardiac cycle, diastole and systole. The change in the ventricular volume from diastole to systole is apparent from images.

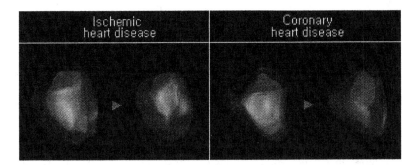

**Fig. 1.** Reconstruction of endo- and epicardial walls using gated SPECT.

## 3   Measuring Diagnostic Data

### 3.1   Diagnostic Data for the Analysis of Ventricular Function

**Ventricular volume:** To study the LV, a cavity volume is an important parameter as well as its temporal evolution. The ventricular volume has been calculated by adding areas of the individual cross sections multiplied by the slice distance between them. In the case of low-resolution images such as SPECT, however, volume calculation based on voxel's size can be over- or underestimated. In our modeling framework, we choose an arbitrary vertex of each face $F_j$ in the model denoted by $P_{Fj}$. The volume inside the model with $m$ faces labeled $F_1, \cdots, F_m$ is given by Eq. (1).

$$V = \frac{1}{3}\sum_{j=1}^{m} P_{Fj} \cdot A_j = \frac{1}{6}\sum_{j=1}^{m} P_{Fj} \cdot (2A_j) \quad \text{where } A_j \text{ is the vector of } F_j \tag{1}$$

**Ejection fraction:** Once we have computed the values of the volume during a cardiac cycle, $EF$ (Ejection Fraction: the percentage of blood that leaves the heart with each beat) can be computed according to the following formula:

$$EF(\%) = \frac{EDV - ESV}{EDV} \times 100 \tag{2}$$

where *EDV* is the LV volume at the end of the diastole and *ESV* is the LV volume at the end of the systole.

**Myocardial mass:** In order to estimate myocardial mass, 1D method such as M-mode method or 2D methods such as area length method and truncated ellipsoid model have been widely used. In our study, both endo- and epicardial surfaces are reconstructed at all time frames and the difference of the volume of epicardial cavity and the volume of endocardial cavity is calculated. Once we calculate the values of endo- and epicardial volumes, we can easily obtain myocardial mass by Eq. (3). The product of the volume of the myocardium and the specific weight of muscle tissue (1.05 g/cm$^3$) gives myocardial mass. It is generally easier to estimate endo- and epicardial volumes at the end of diastole because the ventricular shape tend to be more spherical and smooth with increasing ventricular size. Hence, the end-diastolic frame is usually selected to calculate myocardial mass.

$$1.05 \times \left( \quad EDV \ of \ the \ epicardium \quad - \quad EDV \ of \ the \ endocardium \quad \right) \qquad (3)$$

**Endo- and epicardial wall motions:** In current clinical practice, a semi-quantitative method that derives wall motion score based on a visual impression of regional wall motion is commonly utilized. Here, the averaged wall motion is quantified at twenty-four wall segments. As a practical approach, endo- and epicardial walls can be divided into three equal levels along the apex to base length resulting in its partition into basal, middle, and apical levels. Then each level is divided into eight wall segments. In our study, we can easily observe that the magnitudes of endocardial wall motions are generally larger than those of epicardial wall motions.

**Myocardial wall thickness and thickening:** For wall thickness calculation, a well-known method is 2D centerline method. In this method the wall thickness is computed from endo- and epicardial walls from a single image. However, we calculate wall thickness by using the extended 3D center-surface method. To define a center-surface (a mid-myocardial surface) between endo- and epicardial surfaces, we extract triangle vertices from the both surfaces. Then, each vertex of the endocardial surface is matched to the closest vertex of the epicardial surface. If several vertices of the endocardial surface are matched to the same vertex of the epicardial surface and then averaging is applied and the unmatched vertex of the epicardial surface is matched to the closest vertices of the endocardial surface. Using the estimated center data points, we can reconstruct an estimated center-surface between two cardial surfaces. At a given triangle on the center-surface, two vectors are perpendicular to the surface, and they point endo- and epicardial directions. The wall thickness is computed by summing their lengths (wall thickness = A+B) and the percent increase of wall thickness (wall thickening) is calculated by Eq. (4). If the triangulated surfaces are smooth and the triangles on the surfaces are very small then the line segments A and B have the nearly same vector with different direction. If it is not the case, the wall thickness can be calculated much more robustly by using the present center-surface method.

$$\left[ \left( wall \ thickness_{ES} - wall \ thickness_{ED} \right) / wall \ thickness_{ED} \right] \times 100 \qquad (4)$$

### 3.2 Validation: Ejection Fraction and Myocardial Mass

Several kinds of software [9] for quantification and mathematical models [10,11] have been developed and applied to clinical practice. These include Quantitative Gated SPECT (QGS, Cedars-Sinai Medical Center), the Emory Cardiac Toolbox (ECT; Emory University), 4D-MSPECT (University of Michigan Medical Center), Mathematical Cardiac Torso (MCAT) phantom [10] and NURBS-based phantom [11]. All have correlated well with conventional methods for calculating the ejection fraction. To validate the accuracy of the ejection fraction, our method was compared with the results of the QGS software program using the same images. In our study, the ejection fraction calculated by the QGS (Fig. 2b) showed slightly higher values than did our method (Fig. 2a). However, a good correlation was found between the QGS and our method. It is also clear that our method have the potential to model ventricular shapes more realistically than models based on geometric solids.

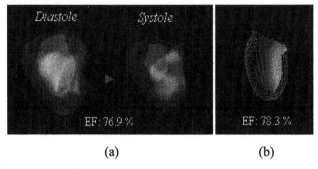

(a)                              (b)

**Fig. 2.** Reconstruction of endo- and epicardial walls: normal subject.

The difference of myocardial mass between time frames would be a good validation check. In our study, the value of *coefficient of variation (CV)* was calculated and compared with the results of the previous studies. The *CV* is a relative measure of variation and is defined as 100 times the ratio of the standard deviation to the mean. The value of the *CV* calculated by our method for the normal subject was 5.0%. This was less than the *CV* calculated by the voxel-based method (*CV* = 6.7%) applied to the same images. We also compared our method with a parametric deformable model based on a superquadric fit followed by free-form deformation (*CV* = 10.5%) [6] and an analytical superellipsoid model widely used in computer vision and graphics to approximate 3D objects (*CV* = 11.8%) [6]. The results indicate that myocardial mass can be measured by our method with reasonable accuracy and it is much more robust than previous methods.

## 4   Visualizing Diagnostic Data Using 3D Glyphs

In this section, we present some ideas on the interactive visualization of diagnostic data described in section 3. A glyph is a graphical object or symbol that represents data through location, size, shape, color or temporal. 2D glyphs have been thoroughly studied and successfully applied to many areas. The meaning of a well-designed glyph is immediately understood by the user without extensive learning. With 3D glyphs, the designer can encode more information with a single glyph than is possible with a 2D glyph [12,13]. Fig. 3 shows some examples of 3D glyphs for time-oriented information (Fig 3a), region-oriented information (Fig 3b) and combined information (Fig 3c), respectively.

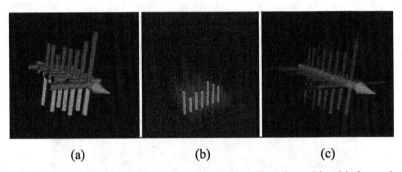

(a)                    (b)                    (c)

**Fig. 3.** 3D glyphs for time-oriented, region-oriented, and combined information.

**Time-oriented information:** A conventional way to visualize time-oriented information involves a time-series plot – a line chart with time on the $x$-axis and a variable on the $y$-axis. Here, the *3D time series spiral glyph* is used to display regional wall motions of the LV over a cardiac cycle. A horizontal arrow shows time and a cylinder bar shows the magnitude of wall motion at each sub-region. Active labels are generated on-the-fly with the exact data for that bar. The 3D time series spiral glyph displays multiple time series at the same time. Moreover it allows user to control the displayed scene by applying interactive filters. Filtered parts of dataset (e.g. small movements (<2.5mm), end-systole or end-diastole) can be selected and displayed in different colors for better interpretation.

**Region-oriented information:** The *3D histogram glyph* is used to display regional wall thickness from apex to the most basal level. Clicking on a part of the *LV-shaped glyph* (as in Fig. 4) selects a single level and the selected level shows up as colored bars within a 3D histogram glyph and the unselected levels are displayed as transparent bars. It also allows dynamic control using filters.

**Combined information:** In order to compare or correlate some data, user can combine clinically useful data into a single 3D glyph (wall thickness at end-systole and at end-diastole, endo- and epicardial wall motions), giving access to several aspects of the data at once. Fig. 3c shows the endo- and epicardial wall motions of the selected sub-region together.

Fig. 4 shows a user interface for 3D glyph-based visualization for multidimensional diagnostic data in cardiology. The introduction of interactive visualization using 3D glyphs with active labels has a positive effect on the interpretation of typical datasets quantitatively and qualitatively. One another advantage of the glyph approach is that its attributes are naturally associated with perceptual elements. For example, a bright color, such as red or yellow, can represent the importance of a data parameter.

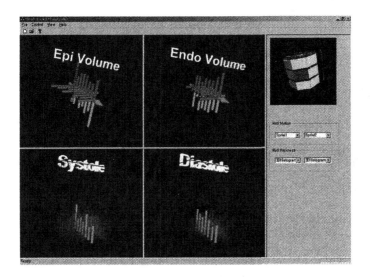

**Fig. 4.** Interactive visualization for multidimensional diagnostic data.

## 5   Conclusions

We have presented information-rich glyphs and applied them to multidimensional diagnostic data from cardiac images, such as wall motion and wall thickness. We also described accurate measurement methods for cardiac diagnosis. As a result of comparing our method with previous studies, we could see a good correlation with respect to ejection fraction. Myocardial mass was measured much more robustly than the previous methods. Besides, glyph-based visualization could allow users to identify and compare some data with easy. This perceptually easy interface can be applied to many diagnostic and patient monitoring applications, such as the evaluation of treatments and precise monitoring of disease progression.

**Acknowledgements.** This work was supported in part by a grant of the Korea Health 21 R&D Project, Ministry of Health & Welfare (02-PJ1-PG3-51312-0003). This work was also supported in part by the Ministry of Science and Technology under the NRL Program.

# References

[1] A. Pentland, B. Horowitz, Recovery of Nonrigid Motion and Structure, IEEE Transactions on Pattern Analysis and Machine Intelligence 13(7) (1991) 730-742.

[2] C.W. Chen, T.S. Huang , M. Arrott, Modelling, Analysis, and Visualization of Left Ventricle Shape and Motion by Hierarchical Decomposition, IEEE Transactions on Pattern Analysis and Machine Intelligence 16(4) (1994) 342-356.

[3] T. McInerney, D. Terzopoulos, A Dynamic Finite Element Surface Model for Segmentation and Tracking in Multidimensional Medical Images with Application to Cardiac 4D Image Analysis, Computerized Medical Imaging and Graphics 19(1) (1995) 69-83.

[4] C. Naster, N. Ayache, Frequency-Based Nonrigid Motion Analysis: Application to Four Dimensional Medical Images, IEEE Transactions on Pattern Analysis and Machine Intelligence 18(11) (1996) 1067-1079.

[5] J. Park, D. Metaxas, L. Axel, Analysis of left ventricular wall motion based on volumetric deformable models and MRI-SPAMM, Medical Image Analysis 1(1) (1996) 53-71.

[6] E. Bardinet, L. D. Cohen, N. Ayache, Tracking and motion analysis of the left ventricle with deformable superquadrics, Medical Image Analysis 1(2) (1996) 129-149.

[7] S.M. Choi, M.H. Kim, Motion Visualization of Human Left Ventricle with a Time-Varying Deformable Model for Cardiac Diagnosis, The Journal of Visualization and Computer Animation 12(2) (2001) 55-66.

[8] S.M. Choi, Y.K. Lee, M.H. Kim, Quantitative Analysis and Visualization of the Endocardial and Epicardial Walls Using Gated SPECT Images, Proceedings of SPIE's International Symposium on Medical Imaging, San Diego, California, USA (2001) 427-435.

[9] K. Nakajima, T. Higuchi, J. Taki, *et al.*, Accuracy of Ventricular Volume and Ejection Fraction Measured by Gated Myocardial SPECT: Comparison of 4 Software Programs, The Journal of Nuclear Medicine 42(10) (2001) 1571-1578.

[10] P.H. Pretorius, W. Xia, M.A. King, *et al.*, Evaluation of Right and Left Ventricular Volume and Ejection Fraction Using a Mathematical Cardiac Torso Phantom, Journal of Nuclear Medicine 38(10) (1997) 1528-1535.

[11] W.P. Segars, D.S. Lalush, B.M.W. Tsui, A realistic spline-based dynamic heart phantom, IEEE Transactions on Nuclear Science 46(3) (1999) 503-506.

[12] F. Oellien, W.D. Ihlenfeldt, Multi-Variate Interactive Visualization of Data from Digital Laboratory Notebooks, ECDL WS Generalized Documents (2001) 1-4.

[13] M. Chuah, S. G. Eick, Information Rich Glyphs for Software Management Data, IEEE Computer Graphics and Applications July/August (1998) 24-29.

# Predicting Influenza Waves with Health Insurance Data

Rainer Schmidt and Lothar Gierl

Universität Rostock, Institut für Medizinische Informatik und Biometrie,
Rembrandtstr. 16 / 17, D-18055 Rostock, Germany
{rainer.schmidt / lothar.gierl}@medizin.uni-rostock.de

**Abstract.** In the recent years, many of the most developed countries have started to develop influenza surveillance systems, because influenza is the last of the classic plagues of the past, which still has to be brought under control and because influenza causes a lot of costs. Efforts have been undertaken on the basis of data from health centres. An alternative is to develop surveillance nets. General practitioners voluntary send reports about the influenza situation in their practise. We have developed a method to predict influenza waves on the basis of health insurance data. In this paper, we introduce different data sources and ideas how to predict influenza waves. We summarise our method, and the main part of the paper deals with first experimental results.

## 1    Introduction

Many people believe influenza to be rather harmless. However, every year influenza virus attacks worldwide over 100 million people [1] and kills alone in the United States between 20.000 and 40.000 people [2]. The most lethal outbreak ever, the Spanish Flu in 1918, claimed 20-40 million lives worldwide, which is more than the second world war on both sides together [3].

Since influenza results in many costs, e.g. for delayed stays in hospital and especially for an increased number of unfitness for work, many of the most developed countries have started to generate influenza surveillance systems (e.g. US: www.flustar.com, France [4], and Japan [5]). The idea is to predict influenza waves or even epidemics as early as possible and to indicate appropriate actions like starting vaccination campaigns or advising high-risk groups to stay at home.

Considerations about how to predict influenza waves begin with questions about which data should be used and which data are available. The answer varies with the country and its health organisation. In countries with rather private health systems like Germany, research groups interested in predicting influenza have often started to develop surveillance nets based on voluntary participation of general practitioners. They felt that the data collected and provided by official health centres were insufficient and often only available with a delay of two or even three weeks. General practitioners usually once a week give some sort of standardised report. Unfortunately, there are some disadvantages. It needs a huge effort to initiate and organise such nets and very often rural areas are not adequately represented, because it is difficult to find doctors willing to participate. Since the reports are always subjective, misjudgements and data interpretation errors may occur, which may lead

P. Perner et al. (Eds.): ISMDA 2003, LNCS 2868, pp. 91-98, 2003.

to false assessments – especially in areas with low density of participating doctors. The alternative means to use official data from health centres. In Germany, these data are more objective, because they contain reports and laboratory results of all occurrences of notifiable diseases. Unfortunately, because of the hierarchical and bureaucratic organisation of the health centres, the availability of these data is delayed for at least two weeks. In countries with more public health systems, sometimes the situation seems to be much better, e.g. in Japan [5].

However, we have chosen another alternative. Since 1997 we receive data for our federal state Mecklenburg-Western Pomerania from the main health insurance scheme. These data are written confirmations of unfitness for work of employees and of people who receive unemployment benefit. Fortunately we get the data daily. Of course there is a short delay between doctors writing the confirmations and the insurance scheme receiving them by mail from their policyholders. We do not recur on the days when the confirmations have been issued by doctors, but on the daily data sets received by the insurance scheme. Since there are some daily fluctuations by chance, so far our prognostic method uses weekly aggregated data. In the future, we hope to refine it to work on a daily basis. The disadvantage of the insurance data is their superficiality, because the confirmations usually contain just the first diagnoses, which might be refined or changed later on. When looking at these data for e.g. salmonellae this is a problem, because usually general practitioners at first just diagnose diarrhoea. However, for influenza this is only a minor problem, because the symptoms of influenza, acute bronchitis, etc. are so similar that most surveillance groups use all acute respiratory diseases to infer influenza.

The next question is "Are data about infected people sufficient to predict influenza waves?" Of course there are a couple of influence factors that might be considered. One of them is the weather. It is assumed that a strong winter increases the spread of influenza. Other factors are the mutations of the virus and influenza outbreaks in foreign countries, even as far as Hongkong. Since no knowledge about these factors is available, all surveillance systems focus on observed numbers of infected people, especially on their increase.

All influenza surveillance systems make use of developments in the past. Most of them have tried statistical methods, so far only with modest results. The usual idea is to compute mean values and standard courses based on weekly incidences of former influenza seasons (from October till March) and to analyse deviations from a statistic normal situation. Influenza waves usually occur only once a season, but they start at different time points and have extremely different intensities. So, Farrington already pointed out that statistical methods are inappropriate for diseases like influenza that are characterised by irregular cyclic temporal spreads [6].

Instead, we have developed a method that uses former influenza seasons more explicitly. We apply the Case-Based Reasoning idea: we determine the most similar former courses of weekly incidences and use them to decide whether a warning is appropriate. Viboud [7] from the group that is responsible for the French Surveillance net has developed a method that is very similar to our one. However, both methods differ in their intentions. Viboud attempts to predict incidences few weeks in advance, while we are interested in more practical results, namely in the computation of appropriate warnings.

## 2    Prognostic Method

Inspired by our former program for the prognosis of kidney function courses [8], we have developed a method to decide about the appropriateness of warnings against approaching influenza waves.

Every influenza season consists of 26 weeks (from October till March). Since we consider weekly incidences, seasons are represented as sequences of 26 numeric values. Each week it has to be decided anew whether a warning is appropriate or not. For this decision, just the recent development is important. So, we consider only a sequence of the four most recent weeks. When an influenza season is finished, it is separated into 23 four-weeks courses; all of them are stored as cases in the case base.

The first step of our method is a temporal abstraction of a sequence of four weekly incidences into three trend descriptions that assess the changes from last week to this week, from last but one week to this week and so forth. Secondly, these three assessments and the four weekly incidences are used to determine similarities between a current query course and all four-weeks courses stored in the case base. Our intention for using these two sorts of parameters is to ensure that a query course and an appropriate similar course are on the same level (similar weekly incidences) and that they have similar changes on time (similar assessments). More details about these first two steps of our method can be found in [9].

The result of computing distances is a very long list of all former four-weeks courses sorted according to their distances in respect to the query course. For the decision whether a warning is appropriate, this list is not really helpful, because most of the former courses are rather dissimilar to the query course. So, the next step means to find the most similar ones. We decided to filter the most similar cases by applying two explicit similarity conditions. First, the difference concerning the sum of the three trend assessments between a query course and a similar course has to be below a threshold X. This condition guarantees similar changes on time. And secondly, the difference concerning the incidences of the current weeks must be below a threshold Y. This second condition guarantees an equal level of the current week of a similar case and the current week of the query course. We have learned good settings for the threshold parameters X and Y by taking in turn one season out of the case base and comparing the results when varying the settings.

The result of this third step usually is a very small list containing only the most similar former courses. As in compositional adaptation [10] we take the solutions of a couple of similar cases into account, namely of all courses in this small list.

In retrospect, we have marked those time points of the former influenza seasons where we believed a warning would have been appropriate; e.g. in the 4th week of 2001, which is the 17th week of the 2000/2001 season (marked as square in fig.1).

For the decision to warn, we split the list of the most similar courses in two lists. One list contains those courses where a warning was appropriate; the second list gets the other ones. For both of these new lists we compute their sums of the reciprocal distances of their courses to get sums of similarities. Subsequently, the decision about the appropriateness of a warning depends on the question which of these two sums is bigger.

## 3    Experimental Results

We have mainly tested our method on health insurance data for the German federal state Mecklenburg-Western Pomerania. Additionally, we applied it on data from a Scottish net of health spotter centres.

### 3.1 Health Insurance Data for Mecklenburg-Western Pomerania

First, we have marked those time points where we, in retrospect, believed a warning would have been appropriate (the three squares in figure 1). Later on we assumed that these warnings might be a bit late. So, we have additionally attempted earlier desired warnings (the three circles in figure 1).

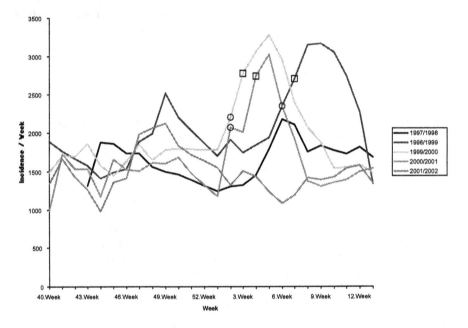

**Fig.1.** Influenza seasons of Mecklenburg-Western Pomerania

### 3.1.1 First Experiment

For our first tests, we used the five seasons shown in figure 1 with the desired warnings depicted as squares. In turn we used one season as query course. Furthermore, we wanted to discover how much the results are improved by the number of seasons stored in the case base. So, for every query season we varied the case base, and we did not only put the seasons in chronological order into the case base, but attempted every combination. That means, for each query season we made four attempts with one season in the case base, six attempts with two seasons etc.

The results are shown in table 1. Sensitivity means proportion of computed warnings to desired warnings; specificity means proportion of computed "non-warnings" to desired "non-warnings". At first glance the results seem to be very good: there are no false warnings and to exactly compute the desired warnings, for every season it is sufficient to use just three of the four remaining seasons as case base. However, since for every query season 23 decisions have to be made, most of them are obvious "non-warnings", a few are follow-up warnings (determined by a simple heuristic when the week before a warning or a follow-up warning was computed), and only few decisions are really crucial.

| | Sensitivity | Specificity |
|---|---|---|
| 1 season in case base | 50 % | 100 % |
| 2 seasons in case base | 83 % | 100 % |
| 3 seasons in case base | 100 % | 100 % |
| 4 seasons in case base | 100 % | 100 % |

**Table 1.** Sensitivity and specificity of our first experiment

### 3.1.2 Earlier Warnings

Since we imagined that the desired warnings of our first experiment might be a bit late, we tried earlier ones in a second experiment, in figure 1 depicted as circles. We made the same experiment again and the results are shown in table 2.

| | Sensitivity | Specificity |
|---|---|---|
| 1 season in case base | 45 % | 95 % |
| 2 seasons in case base | 69 % | 96,7 % |
| 3 seasons in case base | 80 % | 97,2 % |
| 4 seasons in case base | 80 % | 96,1 % |

**Table 2.** Sensitivity and specificity of our second experiment: with earlier warnings

Now it is more difficult to compute the new desired warnings. However, the problems are mainly caused by the peak in the 49th week of 1998, which is the 10th week of the 1998/1999 season. Since the incidences of this peak are higher than the incidences of the desired warnings and the developments are similar too, consequently a warning is computed. Only in retrospect it becomes clear that this was not the beginning of an influenza wave. And since this peak is marked as not worth for a warning, it prevents our program from computing desired warnings for other seasons.

However, this is not so much a problem of the method, but rather a question of the availability of appropriate data. Since we use health insurance data, we do not have access to laboratory results, which often indicate causes. In fact, concerning the analysis of such data by the Robert-Koch Institute [11], the peak in the 49th weak of 1998 was probably (but this was never definitely proved) the result of a pathogen (respiratory syntactical virus) that causes similar symptoms as influenza. Unfortunately, such data from health centres even the Robert-Koch Institute gets only delayed (about two weeks).

### 3.2 Scottish Data from Spotter Centres

Just for experimental reasons we have additionally applied our method on data for Scotland (fig. 2), which we have got from literature [12]. There are seven influenza seasons, two of them with extreme influenza waves, two with rather moderate waves, and three without any noticeable waves.

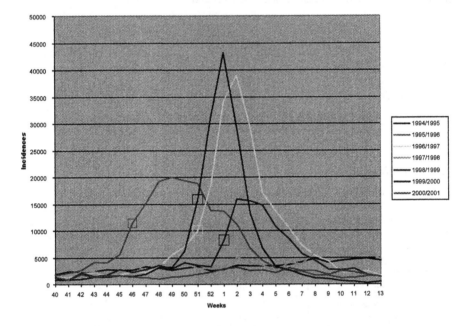

**Fig.2.** Influenza seasons of Scotland

Between figure 1 and figure 2 there are two obvious differences. First, the influenza waves occur earlier in Scotland (already about the turn of the year) than in Mecklenburg-Western Pomerania, and mainly, for this Scottish data influenza waves are more discriminating from "normal" situations.

Here we did not undertake the experiments we have done for Mecklenburg-Western Pomerania, but simply used one season in turn as query course and the remaining six seasons as case base. First, we set the desired warnings as indicated by squares in figure 2. For every season our program computed exactly all desired warnings. It was even possible to obtain this result by using slightly earlier desired warnings, but only as long as these warning situations were discriminating enough from "non-warning" situations.

## 4    Conclusion

In contrast to most medical diagnostic problems, we cannot ask experts about the correctness of the computed warnings. Instead, nobody knows in which week a first warning should be computed. Everybody will agree with "warn as early as possible". But nobody wants too many false warnings.

So far, it is impossible to assess the quality of our method. However, we believe that the results of influenza surveillance depend more on the data than on the method. This does not only mean the a priori quality of the data and the speed of their availability, but additionally the quality for discriminating risky situations. The a priori quality of our health insurance data is rather poor, especially the diagnoses are often superficial, but there is only a very short delay concerning their availability. Official data from German health centres are more profound, but for bureaucratic reasons there availability is delayed for too long.

We do not know anything about the quality and the availability of the Scottish data, except that they are based on data from spotter centres in a country with a rather public health system. However, it is obvious that it is easier to discriminate influenza waves from "normal situations" with this data than with our health insurance data for Mecklenburg-Western Pomerania. Unfortunately, we can only speculate about the reasons. The quality of the data might be better, or the Scottish influenza waves might have been much stronger, or it might even be pure chance. At least such disturbing factors as an occurrence of a virus that has very similar symptoms as influenza is accidental.

# References

1.  Nichol, K.L. et al.: The effectiveness of Vaccination against Influenza in Adults. New England Journal of Medicine 333 (1995) 889-893
2.  Hwang, M.Y.: Do you have the flu? JAMA 281 (1999) 962
3.  Dowdle, W.R.: Informed Consent Nelson-Hall, Inc. Chicago, III
4.  Prou, M., Long, A., Wilson, M., Jacquez, G., Wackernagel, H., Carrat, F.: Exploratory Temporal-Spatial Analysis of Influenza Epidemics in France. In: Flahault, A., Viboud, C., Toubiana, L., Valleron, A.-J.: Abstracts of the 3rd International Workshop on Geography and Medicine, Paris, October 17-19 (2001) 17
5.  Shindo, N. et al.: Distribution of the Influenza Warning Map by Internet. In: Flahault, A., Viboud, C., Toubiana, L., Valleron, A.-J.: Abstracts of the 3rd International Workshop on Geography and Medicine, Paris, October 17-19 (2001) 16
6.  Farrington, C.P., Beale, A.D.:,The Detection of Outbreaks of Infectious Diseases. In: Gierl L. et al. (eds.): International Workshop on Geomedical Systems, Teubner, Stuttgart (1997) 97-117
7.  Viboud, C. et al.: Forecasting the spatio-temporal spread of influenza epidemics by the method of analogues. In: Abstracts of 22nd Annual Conference of the International Society of Clinical Biostatistics, Stockholm, August 20-24 (2001) 71
8.  Schmidt, R., Gierl, L.: Prognoses for Multiparametric Time Courses. In: Brause, R.W., Hanisch, E. (eds.): Medical Data Analysis. Proceedings of ISMDA 2000, Lecture Notes in Computer Science, Vol. 1933, Springer, Berlin Heidelberg New York (2000) 23-33
9.  Schmidt, R., Gierl, L.: Case-Based Reasoning for Prognosis of Threatening Influenza Waves. In: Perner, P. (ed.): Advances in Data Mining. Applications in E-Commerce, Medicine, and Knowledge Management. Lecture Notes in Artificial Intelligence, Vol. 2394, Springer, Berlin Heidelberg New York (2002) 99-107

10.  Wilke, W., Smyth, B., Cunningham, P.: Using Configuration Techniques for Adaptation, In: Lenz, M., et al. (eds.): Case-Based Reasoning Technology, From Foundations to Applications. Lecture Notes in Artificial Intelligence, Vol. 1400, Springer-Verlag, Berlin Heidelberg New York (1998) 139-168

11.  Epidemiologisches Bulletin 18/99, Robert Koch Institute (1999)

12.  Euro surveillance, Vol. 7, No. 12, European Communicable Disease Bulletin (2002) 184-188

# Fuzzy Inference Systems for Multistage Diagnosis of Acute Renal Failure in Children

Marek Kurzynski

Wroclaw University of Technology, Faculty of Electronics, Division of Medical Informatics,
Wyb. Wyspianskiego 27, 50-370 Wroclaw, Poland
kumar@zssk.pwr.wroc.pl

**Abstract.** This paper presents fuzzy inference systems developed for the multistage pattern recognition. Two different methods of generating fuzzy if-then rules from empirical data are presented and their application to the computer-aided diagnosis of acute renal failure are discussed and compared with algorithms based on statistical model.

## 1. Introduction

Designing intelligent diagnostic computer systems has been an important component of research efforts in medical informatics for the last three decades. These systems have been designed to aid physicians to increase their ability and reliability during decision making in diagnosis.

In attempts of algorithmization of medical diagnosis very often formal methods are looked for which could in the best way imitate the natural way of doctor's diagnosis making. As it seems, the process of a doctor making a diagnosis, apart from simple and obvious cases, is a multistage decision one, in which a doctor from stage to stage, as new symptoms are obtained, more accurately determines the patient's pathological condition. The multistage method of pattern recognition can be considered as a formalization of such a sequential decision process and therefore the multistage classifier seems to be a very convenient approach to the problem of computer-aided medical diagnosis.

The paper is a sequel of the author's earlier publications [1,2,3] and it yields new results dealing with the algorithms of multistage recognition for the case when fuzzy inference procedures are applied as diagnostic algorithm.

The contents of the work are as follows. Section 2 describes the multistage classification technique. In Section 3 we introduce necessary background and concepts of different approach to multistage recegnition. In Section 4 fuzzy inference procedure and two methods of deriving the system of fuzzy rules from learning set for particular stages of the multistage pattern recognition are presented. In Section 5 we discuss the results of applications of proposed decision rules to the computer-aided diagnosis of acute renal failure.

P. Perner et al. (Eds.): ISMDA 2003, LNCS 2868, pp. 99-108, 2003.
© Springer-Verlag Berlin Heidelberg 2003

## 2.   Multistage Diagnosis

The procedure in the multistage recognition (diagnosis) consists of the following sequences of activities [2, 3]. At the first stage, some specified symptoms $x_0$ chosen from among all accessible clinical features $x$, describing the patient being diagnosed are measured. These data constitute a basis for making a decision $i_1$. This decision, being the result of diagnosis at the first stage, defines a certain subset in the set of all diseases (states) and simultaneously indicates clinical features $x_{i_1}$ (from among $x$) which should be measured in order to make a decision at the next stage. Now at the second stage, features $x_{i_1}$ are measured, which together with $i_1$ are a basis for making the next diagnosis $i_2$. This diagnosis – like $i_1$ - indicates symptoms $x_{i_2}$ necessary to make the next diagnosis (at the third stage) and – again as at the previous stage – defines a certain subset of diseases, not in the set of all diseases, however, but in the subset indicated by the decision $i_1$, and so one. The whole procedure ends at the last $N$-th stage, where the decision made ( $i_N$ ) indicates a disease unit (a single state), which is the final result of multistage diagnosis. Thus multistage diagnosis means a successive narrowing of the set of potential diseases from stage to stage, down to a disease unit, simultaneously indicating at every stage symptoms which should be measured to make the next diagnosis more precise.

The action of a multistage classifier can be conveniently described by means of a decision-tree (see Fig. 3).

The synthesis of multistage classifier for the computer-aided medical diagnosis is a complex problem. It involves specification of the following components [3]:

* the decision logic, i.e. hierarchical ordering of disease units,
* symptoms (features) used at each stage of diagnosis,
* the decision rules (strategy) for performing the classification.

The present paper is devoted to the last problem only. This means that we shall deal only with the presentation of diagnostic algorithms, assuming that both the tree skeleton and features used at each non-terminal node are specified.

Moreover, our considerations deal with the case when as diagnostic algorithm the fuzzy inference system is applied. Fuzzy systems have successful applications in a wide variety of fields, as for example: automatic control, pattern recognition, signal and image processing, to name only a few. The difference between these systems concentrate on consequences of if-then rules. In accordance with practical requirements and character of considered diagnostic (pattern recognition) problem we assume system with crisp inputs and discrete consequences of rules.

In next section we introduce neccessary notations and present multistage recognition (diagnostic) algorithms under probabilistic model. These algorithms will state conceptual basis for appropriate diagnostic procedures with fuzzy inference engine.

## 3.  Preliminaries and Problem Statement

If we adopt a probabilistic model of the recognition task and assume that the *a priori* probabilities of disease units $p_j$ and conditional probability density functions of symptoms $f_j(x)$ ($x \in X, j \in M = \{1,2,...,M\}$) there exist, then appropriate diagnostic algorithms at particular stages of the classification procedure can be obtained by solving a certain optimization problem. Now, however, in contrast to one-stage recognition, the optimality criterion can be formulated in different ways, and various manners of action of the algorithms can be assumed, which in effect gives different optimal decision rules for the particular stages of classification [3]. Let us consider two cases.

Globally optimal strategy (GOS)

The minimization of the mean probability of misclassification of the whole multistage decision process leads to an optimal decision strategy, whose recognition algorithm at the $n$-th stage is the following [1]:

$$\psi^*_{i_{n-1}}(x_{i_{n-1}}) = i_n \quad \text{if} \tag{1}$$

$$Pc(i_n) \sum_{j \in M_{i_n}} p_j(x_{i_{n-1}}) = \max_{k \in M^{(i_{n-1})}} Pc(k) \sum_{j \in M_k} p_j(x_{i_{n-1}})$$

where $M^{(i_{n-1})}$ denotes the set of decision numbers at the $n$-th stage determined by the decision $i_{n-1}$ made at the previous stage, $M_{i_n}$ denotes the set of class numbers (final diagnoses) accessible after the decision $i_n$ at the $n$-th stage is made. $Pc(i_n)$ is the probability of correct classification at the next stages if at the $n$-th stage decision $i_n$ is made and $p_j(x)$ denotes *a posteriori* probability of disease unit which can be calculated from given data (learning set) using empirical Bayes rule.

What is interesting is the manner of operation of the above decision rule. Namely, its decision indicates this node for which a posteriori probability of set of classes attainable from it, multiplied by the respective probability of correct classification at the next stages of recognition procedure, is the greatest one. In other words, the decision at any interior node of a tree depends on the future to which this decision leads.

Locally optimal strategy (LOS)

Formally, the locally strategy can be derived minimizing the local criteria, which denote probabilities of misclassification for particular nodes of a tree. Its recognition algorithm at the $n$-th stage is the following:

$$\overline{\psi}_{i_{n-1}}(x_{i_{n-1}}) = i_n \quad \text{if} \tag{2}$$

$$\sum_{j \in M_{i_n}} p_j(x_{i_{n-1}}) = \max_{k \in M^{(i_{n-1})}} \sum_{j \in M_k} p_j(x_{i_{n-1}}) .$$

The LOS strategy does not take into regard the context and its decision rules are mutually independent.

In the real world there is often a lack of exact knowledge of *a priori* probabilities and class-conditional probability density functions, whereas only a learning set (the set of case records provided with a firm diagnosis), is known, viz..

$$S = \{(x_1, j_1), (x_2, j_2), ..., (x_L, j_L)\}. \tag{3}$$

In these cases we can to estimate appropriate probabilities and conditional densities from (3) and then to use these estimators to calculate discriminant functions of rules (1) and (2).

In the next section, assuming that the learning set (3) is given, we present the fuzzy inference engine procedure for multistage recognition (diagnosis) and algorithms for the rule system derivation from learning set, which – in some way – correspond to LOS and GOS strategies.

## 4.   Methods

### 4.1.   Diagnostic (Classification) Algorithm

Now we take to decision algorithms for the multistage diagnosis task using the inference engine that makes inferences on a fuzzy rule system. We assume that the form of $k$-th ($k=1,2,...,K$) fuzzy if-then rule at the n-th stage ($n=1,2,..,N$) of recognition (diagnostic) procedure, which associate a diagnosis with an observation (feature) vector

$$x^{(i_{n-1})} = (x_1^{(i_{n-1})}, x_2^{(i_{n-1})}, ..., x_{d_n}^{(i_{n-1})}), \tag{4}$$

is following:

$$IF\ x_1^{(i_{n-1})}\ is\ A_{1,k}\ AND\ x_1^{(i_{n-1})}\ is\ A_{2,k}\ AND...AND\ x_{d_n}^{(i_{n-1})}\ is\ A_{d_n,k}\ THEN\ B_k^{(i_{n-1})}. \tag{5}$$

$A_{i,k}$ denote fuzzy sets (whose membership functions are designated by $\mu_{A_i,k}$) that correspond to the nature of particular observations (for simplicity we assume the sets to be triangular fuzzy numbers) whereas $B$ is a discrete fuzzy set defined on the diagnosis set

$$M^{(i_{n-1})} = \{i_{n-1}^{(1)}, i_{n-1}^{(2)}, ..., i_{n-1}^{(n')}\}, \tag{6}$$

determined by the decision $i_{n-1}$ made at the previous stage, with the $\mu_{B_k}$ membership function.

As diagnostic algorithm the Mamdani fuzzy inference system has been applied [4, 5]. In this system we use the minimum t-norm as AND connection in premises, product operation as conjuctive implication interpretation in rules, the maximum t-conorm as aggregation operation, and finally the maximum defuzzification method. Graphically, applied Mamdani system for two if-then rules, two inputs and discrete conseqence (output) is illustrated in Fig. 1.

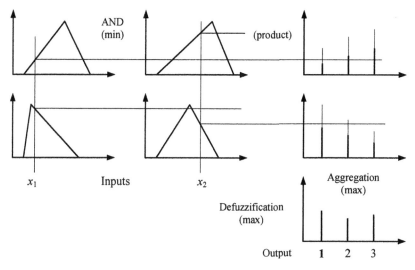

**Fig. 1.** An illustration of the Mamdani fuzzy system with discrete conclusion

## 4.2.  Extraction of Rules

Two methods are used to obtain collection of fuzzy if-then rules (5) in the construction of fuzzy system:
- from human expert or based on domain knowledge,
- extraction of rules using numerical input-output data of the desired system.

One of the best known method of rules generating from the given training patterns, is the method proposed by Wang and Mendel [6] (WM method). This method, developed for the multistage recognition (diagnosis) leads to the following procedure for $i_{n-1}$th node of decision-tree:

1. Divide the spaces of fetures $x_{i_{n-1}}$ into fuzzy regions. In the further example we use triangular fuzzy sets with 3 and 5 partitions as in Fig. 2.

2. For each example generate fuzzy rule with premisses corresponding to fuzzy regions with the highest membership degree of appropriate feature.

3. Find the rules with the same premisses and aggregate them into one rule.

4. Determine the fuzzy conclusion of the rule.

In multistage diagnosis, however, we can in different manner determine the fuzzy conclusion of the rules. Let

$$B_k^{(i_{n-1})} = \{i_{n-1}^{(1)} / \mu_k(i_{n-1}^{(1)}),..., i_{n-1}^{(n')} / \mu_k(i_{n-1}^{(n')})\} \tag{7}$$

be the discrete fuzzy set denotes the conclusion of the $k$-th rule of the system. We propose two different algorithms presented bellow for determining its membership function $\mu$. It leads to the two different fuzzy reasoning systems, which correspond with strategy LOS (2) and GOS (1), respectively.

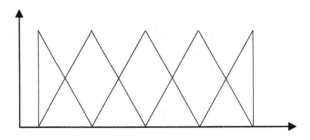

**Fig. 2.** An example of antecedent fuzzy sets with 5 partitions

### 4.2.1.    Algorithm 1
Now

$$\mu_k^{(1)}(i_{n-1}^{(j)}) = \frac{K(i_{n-1}^{(j)})}{\sum\limits_{j=1,2,...,n'} K(i_{n-1}^{(j)})}, \tag{8}$$

where $K(i_{n-1}^{(j)})$ denotes the number of learning patterns fulfiling the $k$-th rule for which the class number is accessible after the decision $i_{n-1}^{(j)}$ at the $n$-th stage is made.

### 4.2.2.    Algorithm 2
Now, to determine membership function of (7), the following formula is proposed:

$$\mu_k^{(2)}(i_{n-1}^{(j)}) = \mu_k^{(1)}(i_{n-1}^{(j)}) \, Pc(i_{n-1}^{(j)}), \tag{9}$$

where $Pc(i_{n-1}^{(j)})$ is the probability of correct classification at the next stages if at the $n$-th stage decision $i_{n-1}^{(j)}$ is made (for the sub-tree with the node $i_{n-1}^{(j)}$ as a root-node.

*Algorithm 1* – similarly as LOS – does not take into regard the context of decision procedure in multistage process, *Algorithm 2*, however, corresponds to the GOS strategy in the probabilistic approch.

In the next section we present results of comparative analysis of proposed algorithms using reach enough set of real-life data that concerns multistage diagnosis of acute renal failure in children.

## 5.    Diagnosis of Acute Renal Failure (ARF) in Children

### 5.1. Material and Diagnostic Problem

ARF is a syndrome of clinical symptoms caused by the adverse action of factors of the urinary tracts. In view of character of the disease a quick and proper diagnosis of ARF is mandatory which is of essential importance for appropriate therapy and prognosis. Unfortunately, the cause of ARF, particularly in the initial phase of the disease is very often difficult to be established, hence a need for computer-aided diagnosis process is clearly evident.

The diagnosis of ARF as a pattern recognition task includes the following 11 classes (etiologic types of ARF) [7]:

| | |
|---|---|
| 1 – toxicosis | 7 – uremic-haemolytic syndrome |
| 2 – nephrotic syndrome | 8 – renal vain thrombosis |
| 3 – sepsis | 9 – andrenogenital syndrome |
| 4 – circulatory failure | 10 – others (intrarenal) |
| 5 – others (prerenal) | 11 – postrenal failure |
| 6 – acute glomerulonephritis | |

The classes have been organized by team of physician into two-stage classifier depicted in Fig. 3.

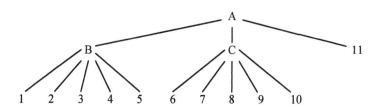

**Fig. 3.** Decision tree for the medical problem in question (A – acute renal failure, B – acute prerenal failure, C – acute intrarenal failure)

Its decision logic (decision tree) is a deliberate one, since from the clinical point of view the most important step is to include the cause of the disease into one of three main categories of ARF and such a partial diagnosis suggests the choice of appropriate therapy.

In the Department of Pediatric Nephrology of Wroclaw Medical Academy the set of 380 case records of children suffering from ARF were collected, which constitute the learning set (3). Each case record contains administrative data, values of 53 clinical features and a firm diagnosis. Most of the diagnoses were made during the period of hospitalization according to the generally accepted criteria. 25 children had died and the anatomopathologic findings provided a definite diagnosis.

Table 1 presents the clinical features collected in case records. We elected to enter into the computer the data, which the registrar obtained at the time when he first saw the case. This is important since clinical data change, and a case which may be extreme puzzling when first seen, may become obvious next morning.

**Table 1.** Clinical features consiered

| |
|---|
| GENERAL |
| Age (1), Weight (2) |
| PHYSICAL EXAMINATIONS |
| Blood pressure – systolic (3), – diastolic (4), Pulse (5), Body temperature (6),.Urine in bladder (7) |
| LABORATORY EXAMINATIONS |
| Sedimentation rate – after 1 hour (8), – after 2 hours (9) |
| GASOMETRIC EXAMINATIONS OF THE BLOOD |
| p $O_2$ (10), p $CO_2$ (11), pH (12), Stand. $HCO_3$ (13), Actual $HCO_3$ (14), BE (15) |
| MORPHOLOGY OF THE BLOOD |
| Leucocytes (16), Reticulocytes (17), Trombocytes (18), Erythrocytes (19), Hemoglobin (20) |
| SERUM |
| Urine level (21), Creatinine level (22), Uric acid level (23), Total protein level (24) |
| SERUM IONOGRAM |
| $Na^+$ (25), $K^+$ (26), $Ca^+$(27) |
| URINE |
| 24-hours amount (28), Specific weight (29), Protein (30), Leucocytes (31), Erythrocytes (32), Protein (33), Cylinders (34) |

## 5.2. Results

First, we have selected the best feature subset for each non-terminal node (the total 34 features were avaliable for selection) using Kolmogorov criterion [8]. Results are listed in Table 2. Each row presents the list of 7 features, selected and ordered according to their Kolmogorov criterion value.

**Table 2.** The results of feature selection

| Node | List of the ranged feature numbers |
|---|---|
| A | 8, 14, 17, 30, 10, 20, 28 |
| B | 29, 6, 24, 5, 15, 22, 32 |
| C | 30, 23, 17, 11, 16, 24, 29 |

In order to study the performance of the proposed recognition concepts and evaluate its usefulness to the computer-aided diagnosis of ARF some computer experiments were made using the leave-one-out method [8]. This method does not require dividing the the data set into learning and testing sets. The leave-one-out method leaves one pattern out of the learning dataset and uses it as a test pattern every time. This procedure continues until each pattern is tested.

At each non-terminal node the features listed in Table 2 were used from the best single one to the set of all 7 features, successively. For fuzzy methods we change also the number of partitions of feature spaces.

Results for probabilistic algorithms LOS and GOS and fuzzy Algorithm 1 and Algorithm 2 are presented in Table 3.

**Table 3.** The results of classification accuracy in percent

| Algorithm | The number of features per node | | | | | | |
|---|---|---|---|---|---|---|---|
| | 1 | 2 | 3 | 4 | 5 | 6 | 7 |
| Probabilistic algorithm LOS | 48.9 | 56.7 | 62.2 | 66.7 | 74.4 | 80.2 | 78.3 |
| Probabilistic algorithm GOS | 47.5 | 56.1 | 64.5 | 69.3 | 77.9 | 87.8 | 84.2 |
| Fuzzy Algorithm 1 (3 partitions) | 45.4 | 54.5 | 61.9 | 70.4 | 78.3 | 75.5 | 70.2 |
| Fuzzy Algorithm 1 (5 partitions) | 47.1 | 55.8 | 62.9 | 73.8 | 80.2 | 77.3 | 72.1 |
| Fuzzy Algorithm 2 (3 partitions) | 47.1 | 57.2 | 63.5 | 71.1 | 81.3 | 79.1 | 70.8 |
| Fuzzy Algorithm 2 (5 partitions) | 48.0 | 58.2 | 65.3 | 74.9 | 84.1 | 80.5 | 73.9 |

These results imply the following conclusions:

1. There occurs a common effect within each algorithm group: algorithms that do not take into regard the context of decision procedure in multistage process (LOS and Algorithm1) are always worse than those that treat multistage procedure as a compound decision process (GOS and Algorithm 2). This confirms the effectiveness and usefulness of the conceptions and algorithm construction principles presented above for the needs of multistage diagnosis.

2. Fuzzy algorithms with 5 partitions of feature spaces are better than algorithms with 3 partitions.

3. The difference between probabilistic algorithms and fuzzy methods is insignificant.

## 6.   Final Remarks

In this paper we focus our attention on the application of a multistage recognition with fuzzy inference system to the diagnosis of acute renal failure. In order to study the performance of the proposed recognition concepts and evaluate its usefulness to the computer-aided diagnosis some computer experiments were made using real data. The objective of our experiements was to measure quality of the tested algorithms that was defined by the frequency of correct decisions.

The comparative analysis presented above for the multistage diagnosis is also of the experimental nature. The algorithm-ranking outcome cannot be treated as one having the ultimate character as a that of a law in force, but it has been achieved for specific data within a specific diagnostic task. However, although the outcome may be different for other tasks, the presented research may nevertheless suggest some perspectives for practical applications.

## Reference

1. M. Kurzynski, Probabilistic Algorithms, Neural Networks, and Fuzzy System Applied to the Multistage Diagnsis of Acute Abdominal Pain, A Comparative Study of Methods, *Proc. 1st Int. Conference on Fuzzy Systems and Knowledge Discovery*, Singapore, 18-20 Nov. 2002 (CD ROM)

2. M. Kurzynski, Multistage Empirical Bayes Approach Versus Artificial Neural Network to the Computer Aided Myocardial Infraction Diagnosis, *Proc. IEEE EMBS Conference*, Vienna, 4-7 Dec. 2002
3. M. Kurzynski, On the Multistage Bayes Classifier, *Pattern Recognition*, vol. 21, pp. 355-365, 1988
4. W. Pedrycz, *Fuzzy Control and Fuzzy Systems*, John Willey & Sons, New York, 1993
5. L-X Wang , *A Course in Fuzzy Systems and Control*, Prentice-Hall, New York, 1998
6. L-X Wang, J.M. Mendel, Generating Fuzzy Rules by Learning from Examples, *IEEE Trans. on SMC*, vol.22, pp. 1414-1427, 1992
7. J. A. James, *Renal Disease in Childhood*, The C.V. Mosby Comp., London, 1996
8. P. Gyorfi, G. Lugossi, *A Probabilistic Theory of Pattern Recognition*, Springer Verlag, New York, 1996

# Data Imbalance in Surveillance of Nosocomial Infections

Gilles Cohen[1], Mélanie Hilario[2], Hugo Sax[3], and Stéphane Hugonnet[3]

[1] Medical Informatics Division, University Hospital of Geneva,
1211 Geneva, Switzerland
Gilles.Cohen@dim.hcuge.ch
[2] Artificial Intelligence Laboratory, University of Geneva,
1211 Geneva, Switzerland
Melanie.Hilario@cui.unige.ch
[3] Department of Internal Medicine, University Hospital of Geneva,
1211 Geneva, Switzerland
{Hugo.Sax,Stephane.Hugonnet@hcuge.ch}

**Abstract.** An important problem that arises in hospitals is the monitoring and detection of nosocomial or hospital acquired infections (NIs). This paper describes a retrospective analysis of a prevalence survey of NIs done in the Geneva University Hospital. Our goal is to identify patients with one or more NIs on the basis of clinical and other data collected during the survey. In this classification task, the main difficulty resides in the significant imbalance between positive or infected (11%) and negative (89%) cases. To remedy class imbalance, we propose a novel approach in which both oversampling of rare positives and undersampling of the non infected majority rely on synthetic cases generated via class-specific subclustering. Experiments have shown this approach to be remarkably more effective than classical random resampling methods.

## 1 Introduction

Surveillance is the cornerstone activity of infection control, whether nosocomial[4] or otherwise. It provides data to assess the magnitude of the problem, detect outbreaks, identify risk factors for infection, target control measures on high-risk patients or wards, or evaluate prevention programs. Ultimately, the goal of surveillance is to decrease infection risk and consequently improve patients' safety. There are several ways to perform surveillance, each method having its advantages and drawbacks. The gold standard is hospital-wide prospective surveillance, which consists in reviewing on a daily basis all available information on all hospitalized patients in order to detect all nosocomial infections. This method is labor-intensive, infeasible at a hospital level, and currently recommended only

---

[4] A nosocomial infection is a disease that develops after a patient's admission to the hospital and is the consequence of treatment—not necessarily surgical—or work by the hospital staff. Usually, a disease is considered a nosocomial infection if it develops 72 hours after admission.

P. Perner et al. (Eds.): ISMDA 2003, LNCS 2868, pp. 109–117, 2003.

for high-risk, i.e., critically ill patients. As an alternative and more realistic approach, prevalence surveys are being recognized as a valid surveillance strategy and are becoming increasingly performed. Their major limitations are their retrospective nature, the dependency on readily available data, a prevalence bias, the inability to detect outbreak (depending on the frequency the surveys are performed), and the limited capacity to identify risk factors. However, they provide sufficiently good data to measure the magnitude of the problem, evaluate a prevention program, and help allocate resources. They give a snapshot of clinically active NIs during a given index day and provide information about the frequency and characterisitics of these infections. The efficacy of infection control policies can be easily measured by repeated prevalence surveys [4].

## 2   Data Collection and Preparation

The University Hospital of Geneva (HUG) has been performing yearly prevalence studies since 1994 [6]. The methodology of prevalence surveys is as follows. The investigators visit all wards of the HUG over a period of approximately three weeks. All patients hospitalized for 48 hours or more at the time of the study are included. Medical records, kardex, X-ray and microbiology reports are reviewed, and additional information eventually obtained by interviews with nurses or physicians in charge of the patient. All nosocomial infections are recorded according to modified Centres for Disease Control (CDC) criteria. Only infections still active at any point during the six days preceding the visit are included. Collected variables include demographic characteristics, admission date, admission diagnosis, comorbidities, McCabe score, type of admission, provenance, hospitalization ward, functional status, previous surgery, previous intensive care unit (ICU) stay, exposure to antibiotics, antacid and immunosuppressive drugs and invasive devices, laboratory values, temperature, date and site of infection, fulfilled criteria for infection. All this information (except those related to infection) are collected for infected and non-infected patients.

Although less time-consuming than prospective surveillance, a prevalence survey nevertheless requires considerable resources, i.e., approximately 800 hours for data collection and 100 hours for entering data in a electronic data base. Due to this important effort, we can afford to perform such studies only once a year. What is particularly time-consuming is the careful examination of all available information for all patients, in order to detect those who might be infected. The aim of this pilot study is to apply data mining techniques to data collected in the 2002 prevalence study in order to detect vulnerability to nosocomial infections on the basis of the factors described above.

The dataset consisted of 688 patient records and 83 variables. With the help of hospital experts on nosocomial infections, we filtered out spurious records as well as irrelevant and redundant variables, reducing the data to 683 cases and 49 variables. In addition, several variables had missing values, due mainly to erroneous or missing measurements. We replaced these missing values with the class-conditional mean for continuous variables and the class-conditional mode for nominal ones.

# 3   The Class Imbalance Problem

The major difficulty inherent in the data (as in many medical diagnostic applications) is the highly skewed class distribution. Out of 683 patients, only 75
(11% of the total) were infected and 608 were not. The class imbalance problem
is particularly crucial in applications where the goal is to maximize recognition
of the minority class[5] The issue of class imbalance has been actively investigated
and remains largely open, but for lack of space we present the major trends very
briefly. The interested reader can refer to [7] for a more comprehensive state of
the art.

   One solution to class imbalance is oversampling the majority class. Typically,
cases from the minority class are replicated until the desired class proportions
are attained. Recently, Chawla et al. [1] replaced straightforward case cloning
by generating synthetic minority class cases from real ones, using a technique
based on nearest neighbors. The opposite approach consists in undersampling,
i.e., subsampling the majority class until its size matches that of the minority
class. Although subsampling is often be done randomly, more guided strategies
have been proposed; for instance, Kubat et al. [9] eliminate redundant, noisy
and borderline cases to downsize the majority class. A third alternative, known
as recognition-based learning, consists in simply ignoring one of the two classes
and learning from a single class; one-class SVMs [10] illustrate this approach
A fourth class of methods involves adjusting misclassification costs: failure to
recognize a positive case (false negative) is penalized more than erroneously
classifying a negative case as positive (false positive) [2]. Contrary to sampling
approaches, cost-based approaches to imbalance involve modifying the learning
algorithm's objective function. However, there are other ways of biasing the
inductive process to boost sensitivity (i.e., capacity to recognize positives). Joshi
et al. [8] decompose set-covering rule induction into a two-stage process: the first
phase maximizes recall of the positive class, while the second phase refines results
of the first phase in order to improve precision.

   In this paper we propose an approach in which **both** oversampling and undersampling (and their combination) are performed using synthetic cases generated in the form of cluster prototypes. The first variant of this approach is
K-means based undersampling of the majority class. This strategy appears unnecessary and even counterintuitive at first sight; one could indeed understandably question the need to generate artificial examples to represent an already
over-represented class. The rationale is that since the artificial examples are built
as centroids of subclusters of the majority class, they thus distill the essential
discriminating properties of that class. For a given cardinality, one could therefore legitimately expect a set of these prototypes to be more informative than a
set of real cases. To shrink the majority class, we ran K-means clustering on the
training instances of this class with $K = N_{min}$, the size of the minority class.
These $N_{min}$ prototypes were then used as sole representatives of the minority

---

[5] For convenience we identify positive cases with the minority and negative cases the
  majority class.

class so that training was performed on equally distributed classes. The second variant involves oversampling the minority class using agglomerative hierarchical clustering (AHC). Partitional clustering methods like K-means are less adequate for this task due to the small number of clusters (and therefore of prototypes) that can be created. The number of clusters K should be considerably less than $N_{min}$; with K=$N_{min}$ each cluster will have a single member which will naturally be its centroid. This is inacceptable since the idea is precisely to synthesize examples that are different from the existing cases (otherwise we revert to standard case duplication). Given this limit on K, the number of synthetic cases generated will be insufficient to attain inter-class equilibrium. Hierarchical clustering does not share this limitation, since the number of (eventually nested) clusters can be augmented at will by increasing the number of levels and varying the inter-cluster distance metrics used. We therefore turned to AHC using single- and complete-linkage in succession to vary the clusters produced. Clusters were gathered from all levels of the resulting dendograms. Their centroids were computed and concatenated with the original positive cases, thus upsizing the positive class to match the negative class. Finally, the third variant is the combination of AHC-based oversampling and K-means based undersampling. Experiments conducted to assess these variants are described in Section 4 and results are discussed in Section 5.

## 4     Experimental Setup

### 4.1     Learning Algorithms

We compared alternative solutions to the class imbalance problem using five learning algorithms with clearly distinct inductive biases. Decision trees such as those built by C4.5 are models in which each node is a test on an individual variable and a path from the root to a leaf is a conjunction of conditions required for a given classification [11]. Naive Bayes computes the posterior probability of each class given a new case, then assigns the case to the most probable class. IB1 is basically a K-nearest-neighbors [3] classification algorithm, while Adaboost builds a single-node decision tree iteratively, focusing at each step on previously misclassified cases [5]. Support vector machines (SVMs) [12] represent a powerful learning method based on the theory of Structural Risk Minimisation (SRM). SVMs learn a decision boundary between two classes by mapping the training data onto a higher dimensional space and then finding the maximal margin hyperplane within that space.

### 4.2     Performance Metrics

In classification tasks, the most commonly used performance metric by far is predictive accuracy. This metric is however close to meaningless in applications with significant class imbalance. To see this, consider a dataset consisting of 5% positive and 95% negatives. The simple rule of assigning a case to the majority class would result in an impressive 95% accuracy whereas the classifier would have failed to recognize a single positive case—an inacceptable situation in medical diagnosis. The reason for this is that the contribution of a class to the overall accuracy rate is a function of its cardinality, with the effect that rare positives have an almost insignificant impact on the performance measure.

To discuss alternative performance criteria we adopt the standard definitions used in binary classification. TP and TN stand for the number of true positives and true negatives respectively, i.e., positive/negative cases recognized as such by the classifier. FP and FN represent respectively the number of misclassified positive and negative cases. In two-class problems, the accuracy rate on the positives, called sensitivity, is defined as $TP/(TP+FN)$, whereas the accuracy rate on the negative class, also known as specificity, is TN/(TN+FP). Classification accuracy is simply $(TP+TN)/N$, where $N = TP+TN+FP+FP$ is the total number of cases.

To overcome the shortcomings of accuracy and put all classes on an equal footing, some have suggested the use of the geometric mean of class accuracies, defined as $gm = \sqrt{\frac{TP}{TP+FN} * \frac{TN}{TN+FP}} = \sqrt{sensitivity * specificity}$. The drawback of the geometric mean is that there is no way of giving higher priority to the rare positive class. In information retrieval, a metric that allows for this is the F-measure $F_\beta = \frac{PR}{\beta P + (1-\beta)R}$, where R (recall) is no other than sensitivity and P (precision) is defined as $P = TP/(TP+FP)$, i.e., the proportion of true positives among all predicted positives. The $\beta$ parameter, $0 < \beta < 1$, allows the user to assign relative weights to precision and recall, with 0.5 giving them equal importance. However, the F-measure takes no account of performance on the negative class, due to the near impossibility of identifying negatives in information retrieval. In medical diagnosis tasks, however, what is needed is a relative weighting of recall and specificity. To combine the advantages and overcome the drawbacks of the geometric mean accuracy and the F-measure, we propose the mean class-weighted accuracy (CWA), defined formally for the K-class setting as $cwa = \frac{1}{\sum_{i=1}^{k} w_i} \sum_{i=1}^{k} w_i accu_i$, where $w_i \in \aleph$ is the weight assigned to class $i$ and $accu_i$ is the accuracy rate computed over class $i$. If we normalize the weights such that $0 \le w_i \le 1$ and $\sum w_i = 1$, we get $cwa = \sum_{i=1}^{k} w_i accu_i$ which simplifies to $cwa = w_i * sensitivity + (1 - w_i) * specificity$ in binary classification.

## 4.3   Evaluation Strategy

The experimental goal was to measure the relative performance of different approaches to adjusting class distribution. Given the limited amount of data, we adopted 5-fold stratified cross-validation in all the experiments. To evaluate our approach, we ran the five learning algorithms (1) on the original class distribution, then on training data balanced via (2) random subsampling,(3) random oversampling, and (4) different variants of our approach as described in Section 3. All learned models were validated on a test set with the original class distribution. In this way, it was ensured that the validation stage was not influenced by any bias introduced by the various class resampling strategies.

## 5   Results

Table 1 summarizes performance results on the original skewed class distribution and illustrates clearly the inadequacy of accuracy for this task. For instance, AdaBoost exhibits the highest accuracy of 90% but actually performs more poorly than Naive Bayes in detecting positive cases of nosocomial infections. In fact, Naive Bayes ranks last in terms of accuracy rate due to its poor performance on the majority class (specificity of 0.88, lower than all the others) but attains the highest sensitivity, 12% higher than that of AdaBoost. Accuracy clearly underestimates the merit of recognizing rare positives.

**Table 1.** Baseline performance (original class distribution: 0.11 pos, 0.89 neg)

| Classifier | Sensitivity | Specificity | CWA | Accuracy |
|---|---|---|---|---|
| IB1 | 0.19 | 0.96 | 0.38 | 0.88 |
| NaiveBayes | 0.57 | 0.88 | 0.65 | 0.85 |
| C4.5 | 0.28 | 0.95 | 0.45 | 0.88 |
| AdaBoost | 0.45 | 0.95 | 0.58 | 0.90 |
| SVM | 0.43 | 0.92 | 0.55 | 0.86 |

We then tested classical methods of random undersampling and oversampling. At each cross-validation cycle, the training set contained 60 positive cases and 486 negative cases. A random sample of 60 negative cases was drawn and used with the 60 available positive cases to train the classifiers. In a separate experiment, positive cases were randomly duplicated until the size of the minority class matched that of the majority class. Table 2 (a) and (b) show performance measures obtained on test data with the original class distribution by classifiers trained on the adjusted class distribution.

**Table 2.** Random subsampling and oversampling (0.5 pos, 0.5 neg)

| (a) Random subsampling | | | | | (b) Random oversampling | | | | |
|---|---|---|---|---|---|---|---|---|---|
| Classifier | Sens | Spec | CWA | Accu | Classifier | Sens | Spec | CWA | Accu |
| IB1 | 0.01 | 0.99 | 0.26 | 0.88 | IB1 | 0.19 | 0.96 | 0.38 | 0.88 |
| NaiveBayes | 0.21 | 0.96 | 0.40 | 0.88 | NaiveBayes | 0.68 | 0.83 | 0.72 | 0.81 |
| C4.5 | 0.00 | 1.00 | 0.25 | 0.89 | C4.5 | 0.49 | 0.87 | 0.59 | 0.83 |
| AdaBoost | 0.04 | 1.00 | 0.28 | 0.89 | AdaBoost | 0.73 | 0.87 | 0.77 | 0.85 |
| SVM | 0.05 | 0.99 | 0.29 | 0.88 | SVM | 0.60 | 0.89 | 0.67 | 0.86 |

The results are contrasted: while random subsampling drastically degraded prediction of positives with respect to the original imbalanced data, random oversampling clearly improved the sensitivity and CWA of all the classifiers except (understandably) IB1. Note that contrary to CWA, accuracy misleadingly decreases with random oversampling.

As explained in Section 3, our approach differs from these random approaches in its principled generation of synthetic samples. In the first variant, we use K-means clustering to subsample the majority class. Results shown in Table 3 (a) support clearly the efficacy of K-means based subsampling. Sensitivity ranges from 0.56 for IB1 to 0.83 and 0.84 for SVM and Adaboost respectively—a visible leap from the 0.19-0.57 interval on the original class distribution and especially from the 0.01-0.21 range attained with random subsampling. More remarkably, specificity did not degrade considerably, so that CWA rates vary between 0.67 and 0.81, definitely better than all previous performance.

**Table 3.** Oversampling and undersampling based on synthetic examples

| (a) K-means subsampling 0.5 pos 0.5 neg | | | | | (b) AHC oversampling 0.38 pos 0.62 neg | | | | |
|---|---|---|---|---|---|---|---|---|---|
| Classifier | Sens | Spec | CWA | Accu | Classifier | Sens | Spec | CWA | Accu |
| IB1 | 0.56 | 0.88 | 0.64 | 0.84 | IB1 | 0.33 | 0.91 | 0.48 | 0.85 |
| NaiveBayes | 0.75 | 0.78 | 0.76 | 0.78 | NaiveBayes | 0.64 | 0.85 | 0.69 | 0.82 |
| C4.5 | 0.72 | 0.67 | 0.71 | 0.68 | C4.5 | 0.45 | 0.87 | 0.56 | 0.83 |
| AdaBoost | 0.84 | 0.74 | 0.81 | 0.75 | AdaBoost | 0.65 | 0.89 | 0.71 | 0.86 |
| SVM | 0.83 | 0.74 | 0.81 | 0.75 | SVM | 0.53 | 0.88 | 0.62 | 0.84 |

We have explained (Section 3) why we chose agglomerative hierarchical clustering to create prototypical instances for oversampling. By combining multilevel clusterings based on single and complete linkage, we were able to compute a total of 234 synthetic instances of the minority class. Added to the 60 original training positives and 486 negatives, they produced a 0.38-0.62 class distribution for training. Results of this operation are shown in Table 3 (b). Here again, sensitivity rates improve significantly over the baseline for all classifiers. However, AHC oversampling improves sensitivity over random oversampling for only 2 out of the 5 classifiers. This can be explained by the fact that in random oversampling positives are as numerous as negatives while they remain outnumbered in 0.38-0.62 AHC distribution.

Finally, we investigated the impact of combining AHC based oversampling and K-means based subsampling. As seen in Table 4, sensitivity and class-weighted accuracy improve over simple AHC oversampling for all classifiers but degrade over K-means subsampling for 4 out of 5 classifiers. For Naive Bayes, however, sensitivity reaches 0.87 and class-weight accuracy 0.84, yielding the maximum performance level recorded over all our experiments.

**Table 4.** Combined AHC oversampling and K-Means subsampling (0.5 pos 0.5 neg)

| Classifier | Sensitivity | Specificity | CWA | Accuracy |
|---|---|---|---|---|
| IB1 | 0.49 | 0.86 | 0.59 | 0.82 |
| NaiveBayes | 0.87 | 0.74 | 0.84 | 0.75 |
| C4.5 | 0.68 | 0.79 | 0.71 | 0.78 |
| AdaBoost | 0.77 | 0.85 | 0.79 | 0.84 |
| SVM | 0.69 | 0.82 | 0.73 | 0.81 |

## 6  Conclusion

We analysed the results of a prevalence study of nosocomial infections in order to predict infection risk on the basis of patient records. The major hurdle, typical in medical diagnosis, is the problem of rare positives. We addressed this problem via a novel approach based on the generation of synthetic instances for both oversampling and undersampling. Generation of artificial cases must however meet a hard constraint: the synthetic cases generated must remain within the frontiers of a given class. This constraint is met by the use of prototypes of class subclusters. Results are indeed promising: whereas the sensitivity range of the 5 classifiers was [0.19-0.57] on the original class distribution, it increased to [0.49-0.87] after combined AHC based oversampling and K-means based subsampling. This suggests that both oversampling and undersampling become more effective when performed using synthetic samples instead of the true instances.

### Acknowledgements

The authors thank Profs. A. Geissbuhler and D. Pittet (University of Geneva Hospitals) for the opportunity to pursue this study.

## References

[1] N. Chawla, K. Bowyer, L. Hall, and W. P. Kegelmeyer. Smote: Synthetic minority over-sampling technique. In *International Conference on Knowledge-Based Systems*, 2000.

[2] P. Domingos. A general method for making classifiers cost-sensitive. In *Proc. 5th International Conference on Knowledge Discovery and Data Mining*, pages 155–164, 1999.

[3] R. Duda, P. Hart, and D. Stork. *Pattern Classification*. Wiley, 2000.

[4] G. G. French, A. F. Cheng, S. L. Wong, and S. Donnan. Repeated prevalence surveys for monitoring effectiveness of hospital infection control. *Lancet*, 2:1021–23, 1983.

[5] Y. Freund and R. E. Schapire. Experiments with a new boosting algorithm. In *Proc. 13th International Conference on Machine Learning*, 1996.

[6] S. Harbarth, Ch. Ruef, P. Francioli, A. Widmer, D. Pittet, and Swiss-Noso Network. Nosocomial infections in swiss university hospitals: a multi-centre survey and review of the published experience. *Schweiz Med Wochenschr*, 129:1521–28, 1999.

[7] N. Japkowicz. The class imbalance problem: A systematic study. *Intelligent Data Analysis Journal*, 6(5), 2002.

[8] M. V. Joshi, R. C. Agarwal, and V. Kumar. Mining needles in a haystack: Classifying rare classes via two-phase rule induction. In *ACM-SIGMOD*, 2001.

[9] M. Kubat and S. Matwin. Addressing the curse of imbalanced data sets: One-sided sampling. In *Procsóf the Fourteenth International Conference on Machine Learning*, pages 179–186, 1997.

[10] L. M. Manevitz and M. Youssef. One-class SVMs for document classification. *Journal of Machine Learning Research*, 2, December 2001.

[11] J. R. Quinlan. *C4.5: Programs for Machine Learning*. Morgan Kaufmann, San Mateo, CA, 1993.

[12] V. Vapnik. *Statistical Learning Theory*. Wiley, 1998.

# An Outline of an Expert System for Diagnosis and Treatment of Bronchogenic Carcinoma*

I. Rodríguez-Daza[1], L.M. Laita[1], E. Roanes-Lozano[2],
A.M. Crespo-Alonso (MD)[3], V. Maojo (MD, PhD)[1], L. de Ledesma[1], and
L. Laita[4]

[1] Universidad Politécnica de Madrid, Dept. of Artificial Intelligence,
Campus de Montegancedo, Boadilla del Monte, 28660-Madrid, Spain
indalord@navegalia.com, {laita,maojo,ledesma}@fi.upm.es
[2] Universidad Complutense de Madrid, Dept. of Algebra,
c/ Rector Royo Villanova s/n, 28040-Madrid, Spain
eroanes@mat.ucm.es
[3] Hospital Virgen de la Salud, c/ Forjadores 2, 45002-Toledo, Spain
anamca@vodafone.es
[4] Universidad Complutense de Madrid, Nursing School,
Ciudad Universitaria, 28040-Madrid, Spain

**Abstract.** We present in this paper a "rule based knowledge system"
for diagnosis and treatment of bronchogenic carcinoma. The rule based
knowledge system consists of a "knowledge base", an "inference engine"
and a "graphical user interface". For the sake of space, these three items
will be described but not completely detailed here. The system is wholly
described in the monograph [14] (in Spanish). The knowledge base contains the experts' knowledge in form of logical expressions. The inference
engine is a program that both verifies consistency of the knowledge base
and extracts automatically consequences from the information used in
building the knowledge base. The latter is implemented in the computer
algebra language CoCoA and is based on a theory original of the team
to which the authors belong. As the paper is intended for different audiences, this theory will be informally presented. A friendly graphical user
interface facilitates the introduction of medical data.

## 1 Introduction and Background

We present in this paper a "rule based knowledge system" (to be denoted RBKS)
for diagnosis and treatment of bronchogenic carcinoma [2, 3, 11, 18, 19].

As most RBKS, ours has three components: a "knowledge base" (denoted
"KB"), an "inference engine" (denoted "IE") and a "graphical user interface"
(denoted "GUI"). For the sake of space, in the present paper we describe these
three items only partly. The system is wholly described (in Spanish) in the
monograph [14].

---

* Partially supported by projects TIC2000-1368-C03-01 and TIC2000-1368-C03-03
(Ministry of Science and Technology, Spain).

P. Perner et al. (Eds.): ISMDA 2003, LNCS 2868, pp. 118–126, 2003.

The KB contains the experts' knowledge in form of condensed expressions (bivalued logical expressions in our case).

The IE is a program that both verifies the consistency of the KB and extracts automatically consequences from the information in the KB. In our case, such program has been implemented in the computer algebra language CoCoA[5] [5, 13]. This implementation is based on a theory, original of the team to which the authors belong. As the paper is intended for different audiences, this theory will be informally presented.

The GUI is a tool that enables users not familiar to computers to introduce data and perform computations easily. In this RBKS the user (a physician) has to choose the corresponding no/yes options (i.e., the data corresponding to the patient) in a windows-style environment. The interface consists of eight screens, being the last one the medical record and diagnosis of the patient.

As we believe that RKBS for diagnosis and treatment in medicine cannot substitute a specialist or a team of specialists, our system has been designed to be no more than a helpful tool for family doctors and specialists. Nevertheless, its use may have advantages because:

1. it may help specialists by contrasting the "opinions" (the outputs) of the RKBS with their own opinions
2. its IE is efficient and, above all, its logic reasoning is exact.

Our logic-mathematical theory, founded on "normal forms" and "Gröbner bases" [1, 17], has as background the works of Kapur and Narendran [8]; Hsiang [7]; Alonso, Briales, Riscos and Chazarain [6] and our work on the application of Gröbner Bases to automated deduction [9, 15], which we applied to the study of medical appropriateness criteria [10], to the diagnosis of anorexia [12] and to other fields (railway interlockings) [16].

The best known related work on RBKS applied to medicine is Buchanan and Shortliffe's classical work [4].

## 2    The Knowledge Base

### 2.1    Production Rules and Facts

Our KB consists logical formulae like:

$$\neg X[1] \wedge \neg X[2] \wedge X[3] \wedge \neg X[4] \rightarrow X[5]$$

These type of formulae are called "production rules". This one is read as follows:

IF not-$X[1]$ and not-$X[2]$ and $X[3]$ and not-$X[4]$ THEN $X[5]$ .

---

[5]  CoCoA, a system for doing Computations in Commutative Algebra. Authors: A. Capani, G. Niesi, L. Robbiano. Available via anonymous ftp from: cocoa.dima.unige.it

The symbols as $X[1]$ and their negations, $\neg X[1]$, are called "literals". $X[1]$ is an example of "variable" (our RBKS contains 160 different variables).

The symbol "$\wedge$" translates "and" and the symbol "$\rightarrow$" translates "implies". Most production rules in this paper have this form; nevertheless, in some cases, a prior grouping of subsets of rules makes the symbol "$\vee$" (meaning "or") to appear intermixed with "$\wedge$".

The set of all literals that appear on the left-hand side of any production rule but not in any right-hand side, together with the set of their contrary literals (say, $X[1]$ is the contrary of $\neg X[1]$ and conversely) is called the "set of potential facts" (to be denoted "SPF").

The user of our expert system, by asking questions to the patient and from the consideration of laboratory and radiological results, builds a "maximal consistent set of potential facts" (one for each patient). This means that the user chooses one and only one element of each pair of the set of pairs in the SPF (there are 77 different pairs). "Consistent" means precisely that never two contrary literals can be chosen for a same patient.

## 2.2    Construction of the KB

Consultation with experts and the literature led us to build several tables of medical practice for diagnosis and treatment of bronchogenic carcinoma. The information contained in those tables (expressed in natural language as statements of the form "IF such fact AND such fact occur THEN such conclusion follows"), was classified under 11 titles and translated into 101 production rules.

For the sake of space we mention only three titles below (the 1st, 2nd and 11th), including only one "IF-THEN" English expression in each of them; together with the corresponding production rule and the translation of the latter to its "prefix form" (as CoCoA requires). In the original work, a list of all 160 RBKS variables with their respective meaning is supplied before listing the production rules.

– Title 1: Consequences of the observation of the thorax X-ray plates.

  • IF-THEN statement #5:    IF a pancoast tumor is observed AND its position is central THEN perform a biopsy by fibrobronchoscopy
  • Production rule R5:    $X[2] \wedge X[8] \rightarrow X[11]$
  • CoCoA input for R5:    `R5:=IMP(AND1(x[2], x[8]), x[11]);`

– Title 2: Study of benignity or malignity.

  • IF-THEN statement #11:    IF pulmonar nodule has a clear-cut margin AND satellite injuries have been produced AND according to prior X-ray plates the nodule size had not changed in the last two years AND its size has doubly increased in the last month THEN benignity criterium II holds.
  • Production rule R11:    $X[138] \wedge X[139] \wedge \neg X[136] \wedge X[137] \rightarrow X[140]$

- CoCoA input for R11:  `R11:=IMP(AND1(AND1(AND1(x[138], x[139]), NEG(x[136])), x[137]), x[140]);`

- Title 11: study of appropriateness of performing surgery.

  - IF-THEN statement #98:   IF patient has (an hamartoma OR a carcinoid) AND he/she fits the pre-surgery criteria THEN perform a carcinoma resection
  - Production rule R98:   $(X[120] \lor X[121]) \land X[133] \rightarrow X[107]$
  - CoCoA input for R98:
    `R98:=IMP(AND1(OR1(x[120], x[121]), NEG(x[133])), x[107]);`

## 3   The Inference Engine

The construction of the IE requires:

1) translating the production rules of the RBKS into polynomials
2) building, from these polynomials, some sets of algebraic expressions (three in our case, I, J and K), called "ideals" and
3) applying to these constructs just two commands of CoCoA: `GBasis(I+K+J)` and `NF(NEG(A₀),I+K+J);` (`GBasis` and `NF` mean Gröbner basis and normal form, respectively).

It is recommended to read the next three subsections while looking in parallel at Section 5 (which contains the corresponding CoCoA procedures).

### 3.1   Translating Production Rules into Polynomials

The expressions of the polynomials corresponding to the four basic bivalued logical formulae (those corresponding to the symbols $\neg, \lor, \land$ and $\rightarrow$) are provided. The uppercase letters represent the variables that stand in the production rules and the lowercase letters represent the corresponding polynomial variables:

- the logical formula *not* $X_1$ ($\neg X_1$) is translated into the polynomial $1 + x_1$
- the logical formula $X_1$ *or* $X_2$ ($X_1 \lor X_2$) is translated into the polynomial $x_1 \cdot x_2 + x_1 + x_2$
- the logical formula $X_1$ *and* $X_2$ ($X_1 \land X_2$) is translated into the polynomial $x_1 \cdot x_2$
- the logical formula $X_1$ *implies* $X_2$ ($X_1 \rightarrow X_2$) is translated into the polynomial $x_1 \cdot x_2 + x_1 + 1$ .

The corresponding CoCoA commands in Section 5 are: `NEG`, `OR1`, `AND1` and `IMP`.

## 3.2    The Ideals I, J, and K

The polynomials we deal with form what algebraists call a "commutative rings with unit". For readers not familiar with algebra, it is enough to say that such structure is a set of polynomials where the two usual operations (sum and product) satisfy some properties (such as the commutative property of the sum: for any polynomials $p$ and $q$ in the ring: $p + q = q + p$). The polynomial ring is declared in the IE through the CoCoA commands in lines 1 and 2 of Section 5.

An ideal is a subset of the commutative ring, which also happens to be a ring, and has the property that the product $i \cdot r$ of any element $i$ of the ideal by any element $r$ of the ring always belongs to the ideal. Subsequently, if the element 1 belongs to the ideal, the ideal is the whole ring.

The ideal "generated" by a set of polynomials in a polynomial ring is the set of polynomials formed by performing sums of products of "generators" by elements in the ring (that is the minimum ideal that contains the "generators").

Let us return to our RBKS. The ideal I is generated by the polynomials of the form $x^2 - x$ and it has the effect of simplifying the polynomials that translate the KB. For instance, x[1]^2-x[1], is the way $x_1^2 - x_1$ is written in CoCoA (see the third line of code in Section 5).

The SPF consists of 77 variables together with their corresponding 77 negations. As said in Section 2, each patient is characterized by a maximal consistent subset of the SPF. Each of these sets generate an ideal, different for each patient. K represents the ideal generated by the facts that characterize a certain patient. The objects that generate K are of the form NEG(F) or NEG(FN), where NEG is required by Theorem 1 below; F is an affirmed fact and FN is a negated fact (see Section 5).

The set of (the polinomial form of the negations of) all the 101 production rules of our KB, denoted as R1, R2,..., R101, generate an ideal which we denote as J (see Section 5).

## 3.3    The Commands GBasis and NF

**Theorem 1.** *A formula $A_0$ "follows" from the formulae in the union of the two sets of formulae:*

$$\{A_1, A_2, ..., A_m\} \cup \{B_1, B_2, ..., B_k\}$$

*that, respectively, represent a maximal consistent subset of the set of potential facts and the set of all production rules of a RBKS if and only if the polynomial translation of the negation of $A_0$ belongs to the ideal I+K+J (generated by the polynomials $x_1^2 - x_1, x_2^2 - x_2, ..., x_n^2 - x_n$ and the polynomial translation of the negations of $A_1, A_2, ..., A_m$ and by the polynomial translation of the negations of $B_1, B_2, ..., B_k$).*

In this RBKS, I and J are fixed, meanwhile K depends on the patient considered. Regarding $A_0$, it can be either a diagnosis or a treatment.

That $A_0$ follows from the formulae in $\{A_1, A_2, ..., A_m\} \cup \{B_1, B_2, ..., B_k\}$ is checked in CoCoA by typing:

```
NF(NEG(A[0]),I+K+J);
```

If the output is 0, the answer is "yes"; if the output is different from 0, the answer is "no".

A RBKS is inconsistent if a contradiction is a consequence of the information contained in the RBKS.

Inconsistency is expressed by the algebraic fact that I+K+J degenerates into the whole ring , i.e. that 1 belongs to I+K+J. This condition can be checked by typing in CoCoA:

```
GBasis(I+J+K);
```

If the output is 1 (it appears as [1] on the CoCoA screen), the RBKS is inconsistent; otherwise, the RBKS is consistent (in this case the output is usually a large set of polynomials).

## 4    Diagnoses and Treatments of Bronchogenic Carcinoma

The characteristics of each patient have to be chosen from the 77 pairs of potential facts. For the sake of space, only 11 of them are listed below:

- condensation = yes, $x[6]$
- carcinoma peripherial position = yes, $x[9]$
- peripheral arteriopathy = yes, $x[7]$
- biopsy detects cancer cells = yes, $x[19]$
- carcinoma compatible with adenocarcinoma = yes, $x[29]$
- invasion of main bronchio farther than 2 centimeters of the carine = yes, $x[44]$
- athelectasia = no, $\neg x[115]$
- malignant pleural overflow = no, $\neg x[50]$
- craneal TC test positive = no, $\neg x[64]$
- Kamofsky > 40 = no, $\neg x[90]$
- PaCO2 < 45 mg = no, $\neg x[95]$.

The ideal K corresponding to this patient is then constructed (see Section 5).

As illustration, we can now ask (for such a patient): **Perform lobectomy?** (to which variable $x[103]$ was assigned):

```
NF(NEG(x[103]), I+K+J);
```

The output is "0", which means "**yes**", lobectomy ought to be performed.

Many other questions as whether to apply radiotherapy or quimiotherapy or not, the state on which the illness is, etc. can be asked to the system in a similar way.

# 5   CoCoA Implementation of the Inference Engine

- Definition of the ring, the ideal I and the polynomial translation of the logical operations:

```
A ::=Z/(2)[x[1..160]];
USE A;
I:=Ideal( x[1]^2-x[1], ..., x[160]^2-x[160] );
NEG(M):=NF(1+M,I);
OR1(M,N):=NF(M+N+M*N,I);
AND1(M,N):=NF(M*N,I);
IMP(M,N):=NF(1+M+M*N,I);
```

- The 101 production rules should be entered now (see Section 2.2).
- The SPF should be entered next:

```
F1:=x[1];          F1N:=NEG(x[1]);
F2:=x[2];          F1N:=NEG(x[1]);
   ...                 ...
```

- Definition of the ideals J and K:

```
J:=Ideal( NEG(R1),NEG(R2), ..., NEG(R101) );
K:=Ideal( NEG(F1),NEG(FN2),NEG(FN34), ... );
```

- Consistency checking

```
GBasis(I+K+J);
```

- Knowledge extraction:

```
NF(NEG(x[103]), I+K+J);
```

# 6   Conclusions

We have presented in outline a RBKS for automated diagnosis and decision taking about treatments for bronchogenic carcinoma. Obviously the goal is not to substitute the specialist, but to help him/her through the comparison of his/her diagnosis with that suggested by the system.

As known from previous research projects in the field since the 70s and 80s [4], knowledge acquisition from experts in a specific domain is a difficult issue. Given the differences in cognitive reasoning and problem solving approaches among across disciplines, communication between medical experts and professionals of other areas is proven to be complex. In this case, to translate medical knowledge into logical format is an additional task to resolve.

The goal of this project is to address for the formalization of a medical domain and to introduce a logic and computer algebra-based approach to medical diagnosis and management. Since medical scientific knowledge is incomplete and clinical interpretations are subjective by nature, our approach aims to expand research in the area of decision supports. Clinical applications of the proposed system should include a comprehensive validation of the tools and knowledge described in this paper.

# References

[1] W.W. Adams, P. Loustaunau, An Introduction to Gröbner Bases (Graduate Studies in Mathematics, American Mathematical Society, Providence, RI, 1994).

[2] American Thoracic Society & European Respiratory Society, Pretreatment evaluation of non-small-cell lung cancer. Am. J. Respir. Crit. Care Med. 156 (1997) 320-332.

[3] J. Baladrón, Neumología y Cirugía Torácica. Curso intensivo MIR Asturias (SL, Oviedo, 1999).

[4] B. Buchanan, E.H. Shortliffe (Editors), Rule Based Expert Systems: the MYCIN Experiments of the Stanford Heuristic Programming Project (Addison Wesley, New York, 1984).

[5] A. Capani, G. Niesi, CoCoA User's Manual v. 3.0b (Dept. of Mathematics - University of Genova, Genova, 1996).

[6] J. Chazarain, A. Riscos, J.A. Alonso, E. Briales, Multivalued Logic and Gröbner Bases with Applications to Modal Logic, J. Symb. Comp. 11 (1991) 181-194.

[7] J. Hsiang, Refutational Theorem Proving using Term-Rewriting Systems, Art. Intell. 25 (1985) 255-300.

[8] D. Kapur, P. Narendran, An Equational Approach to Theorem Proving in First-Order Predicate Calculus (General Electric Corporate Research and Development Report 84CRD296, Schenectady, NY, March 1984, rev. December 1984). Also in: Proceedings of IJCAI-85 (1985) 1446-1156.

[9] L.M. Laita, E. Roanes-Lozano, L. de Ledesma, J. A. Alonso, A Computer Algebra Approach to Verification and Deduction in Many-Valued Knowledge Systems, Soft Comp. 3/1 (1999) 7-19.

[10] L.M. Laita, E. Roanes-Lozano, V. Maojo, L. de Ledesma, L. Laita, An Expert System for Managing Medical Appropriateness Criteria Based on Computer Algebra Techniques, Comp. Math. Appl. 42/12 (2001) 1505-1522.

[11] A. López-Encuentra , M.J. Linares-Asensio, Carcinoma Broncogénico. Pautas de Práctica Clínica en Neumología (Idepsa, Madrid, 1996) 177-185.

[12] C. Pérez. L.M. Laita, E. Roanes-Lozano, L. Lázaro, J. González, L. Laita, A Logic and Computer Algebra-Based Expert System for Diagnosis of Anorexia, Math. Comp. Simul. 58 (2002) 183-202.

[13] D. Perkinson, CoCoA 4.0 Online Help-electronic file acompanying CoCoA v.4.0 (2000).

[14] I. Rodríguez Daza, L. M. Laita, Desarrollo y verificación de un sistema experto para el diagnóstico y clasificación de los tumores broncogénicos, Ltd. dissertation, Facultad de Informática, Universidad Politécnica de Madrid (2002).

[15] E. Roanes-Lozano, L.M. Laita, E. Roanes-Macías, A Polynomial Model for Multivalued Logics with a Touch of Algebraic Geometry and Computer Algebra, Math. Comp. Simul. 45/1 (1998) 83-99.

[16] E. Roanes-Lozano, E. Roanes-Macías, Luis M. Laita, Railway interlocking systems and Gröbner bases, Math. Comp. Simul. 51/5 (2000) 473-481.

[17] F. Winkler, Polynomial Algorithms in Computer Algebra (Springer-Verlag, Vienna, 1996).

[18] –, Protocolo de actuación en tumor pulmonar (Servicio de Neumología, Hospital Virgen de la Salud, Toledo, not dated).

[19] –, Normativa SEPAR sobre Diagnóstico y estadificación del Carcinoma Broncogénico (Sociedad Española de Neumología y Cirugía Torácica, Madrid, 1996). See also: www.separ.es

# Author Index

# Lecture Notes in Computer Science

For information about Vols. 1–2765
please contact your bookseller or Springer-Verlag